Improving Healthcare Using Toyota Lean Production Methods

46 Steps for Improvement

Also available from ASQ Quality Press:

Lean-Six Sigma for Healthcare: A Senior Leader Guide to Improving Cost and Throughput
Chip Caldwell, Jim Brexler, and Tom Gillem

The Manager's Guide to Six Sigma in Healthcare: Practical Tips and Tools for Improvement
Robert Barry and Amy C. Smith

Nan: A Six Sigma Mystery
Robert Barry

Measuring Quality Improvement in Healthcare: A Guide to Statistical Process Control Applications
Raymond G. Carey, PhD and Robert C. Lloyd, PhD

The Six Sigma Book for Healthcare: Improving Outcomes By Reducing Errors
Robert Barry, PhD, Amy Murcko, APRN, and Clifford Brubaker, PhD

Improving Healthcare with Control Charts: Basic and Advanced SPC Methods and Case Studies
Raymond G. Carey

The Six Sigma Journey from Art to Science
Larry Walters

Six Sigma for the Office: A Pocket Guide
Roderick A. Munro

Defining and Analyzing a Business Process: A Six Sigma Pocket Guide
Jeffrey N. Lowenthal

Customer Centered Six Sigma: Linking Customers, Process Improvement, and Financial Results
Earl Naumann and Steven H. Hoisington

Office Kaizen: Transforming Office Operations into a Strategic Competitive Advantage
William Lareau

To request a complimentary catalog of ASQ Quality Press publications, call 800-248-1946, or visit our Web site at http://qualitypress.asq.org.

Improving Healthcare Using Toyota Lean Production Methods

46 Steps for Improvement

Second Edition

Robert Chalice

ASQ Quality Press
Milwaukee, Wisconsin

American Society for Quality, Quality Press, Milwaukee 53203
© 2007 American Society for Quality
All rights reserved. Published 2007
Printed in the United States of America

12 11 10 09 08 07   5 4 3 2

Library of Congress Cataloging-in-Publication Data

Chalice, Robert.
 Improving healthcare using Toyota lean production methods : 46 steps for improvement /
Robert Chalice. — 2nd ed.
   p. ; cm.
 Rev. ed. of: Stop rising healthcare costs using Toyota lean production methods.   2005.
 Includes bibliographical references and index.
 ISBN 978-0-87389-713-6 (pbk. : alk. paper)
  1. Medical care—Cost control. 2. Medical care—Quality control. 3.   Medical care—
Cost effectiveness. 4. Production management. 5. Production control.   I. Chalice, Robert.
Stop rising healthcare costs using Toyota lean production methods. II. American Society for
Quality. III. Title.
  [DNLM: 1. Toyota Jidosha Kabushiki Kaisha. 2.   Health Care Costs—United States.
3.   Cost Control—methods—United States. 4.   Health Care Reform—economics—United
States. 5.   Quality of Health Care—economics—United States.   W 74 AA1 C436s 2007]
  RA410.53.C43 2007
  338.4'33621—dc22   2007004991

ISBN-13: 978-0-87389-713-6

Publisher: William A. Tony

Acquisitions Editor: Matt Meinholz

Project Editor: Paul O'Mara

Production Administrator: Randall Benson

ASQ Mission: The American Society for Quality advances individual, organizational, and
community excellence worldwide through learning, quality improvement, and knowledge
exchange.

Attention Bookstores, Wholesalers, Schools, and Corporations: ASQ Quality Press books,
videotapes, audiotapes, and software are available at quantity discounts with bulk purchases
for business, educational, or instructional use. For information, please contact ASQ Quality
Press at 800–248–1946, or write to ASQ Quality Press, P.O. Box 3005, Milwaukee, WI
53201–3005.

To place orders or to request a free copy of the ASQ Quality Press Publications Catalog,
including ASQ membership information, call 800–248–1946. Visit our Web site at
www.asq.org or http://qualitypress.asq.org.

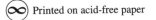 Printed on acid-free paper

Quality Press
600 N. Plankinton Avenue
Milwaukee, Wisconsin 53203
Call toll free 800-248-1946
Fax 414-272-1734
www.asq.org
http://www.asq.org/quality-press
http://standardsgroup.asq.org
E-mail: authors@asq.org

Contents

Preface .... *xi*

Acknowledgments .... *xiii*

Part I U.S. Healthcare System Problems and Solutions 1

Chapter 1   U.S. Healthcare System Problems 3

Rising Health Insurance Premiums 3

Why Double-Digit Health Insurance Increases? 9

46.6 Million Americans (Almost 1 in 6) Are Without
Health Insurance 13

Motivating Healthcare Providers to Reduce Cost and
Improve Quality 15

Toyota Lean Production 18

Waste in Healthcare 21

Excess Healthcare Administrative and Overhead Costs 22

Excess Insurance Company Administrative and
Overhead Costs 26

U.S. Health Expenditures Are a Growing Percentage
of GDP 30

U.S. Spends Twice as Much on Healthcare But Ranks
37th in Health System Performance 32

Quality Problems in U.S. Healthcare 34

Past Failure of Continuous Quality Improvement and Total
Quality Management 38

Redesigning the U.S. Healthcare System 39

Chapter 2   Respect for Employees **41**

**Part II   Reduce Healthcare Cost and Improve Quality
by Using Toyota Lean Production Methods** **43**

**Chapter 3   46 Steps to Improve Cost and Quality in the
U.S. Healthcare System** **45**

Step 1   Define value from the perspective of the
patient (customer)   46

Step 2   Map the patient's value stream   47

Step 3   Walk through all your core processes, and observe
how they work in detail   48

Step 4   Implement Toyota-style lean production
methods   50

Step 5   Train administrators, managers, and supervisors
to be lean leaders   52

Step 6   Provide empathetic "change management" to ease
the transition to lean   55

Step 7   Change "quality improvement department" to "quality
and cost improvement department"   56

Step 8   Change the name "quality improvement manual" to
"quality and cost improvement manual"   57

Step 9   Educate every employee about the basic strategic
plan of the organization   57

Step 10   Establish an improvement plan with goals to be
accomplished by specific people and dates   59

Step 11   Implement a simple scorecard for the entire healthcare
organization   61

Step 12   Use a simple scorecard to monitor each
department   63

Step 13   The board of directors initiates selected strategic
quality and cost improvement goals   65

Step 14   Publish an annual quality report for simultaneous
review with the annual financial report   66

Step 15   Create a rapid improvement team (RIT) to make
quick cost and quality improvements   67

Step 16   Encourage RIT members to implement Toyota-style
work teams   70

Step 17   Implement rapid improvement circles of
employees (RICs)   74

Step 18   Implement a permanent organizational structure for
quality and cost improvement   77

Step 19	Set a goal for each RIC member to produce one to four new suggestions per month	77
Step 20	Have a clear reward and recognition program, and communicate negative consequences	79
Step 21	Adopt and teach continuous improvement to as many people as possible in the organization	79
Step 22	The rapid improvement team quickly implements a 5S program	80
Step 23	Identify unnecessary items using red tags	83
Step 24	Promote visual control throughout the workplace and organization	83
Step 25	Eliminate all forms of waste	85
Step 26	Reduce specific examples of potential waste	103
Step 27	Sequence work and standardize it	109
Step 28	Eliminate bottlenecks to improve continuous flow	110
Step 29	Document all important processes in the organization or department	112
Step 30	Implement and maintain continuous improvement	113
Step 31	Consider radical improvement where appropriate	114
Step 32	Videotape each step of entire work processes	115
Step 33	Use flowcharts to improve core processes	116
Step 34	Use spaghetti diagrams to trace the path of a patient, employee, or product	117
Step 35	Measure process cycle times	117
Step 36	Implement quick changeovers within a process . . .	118
Step 37	Complement nursing care delivery models with Lean	119
Step 38	Challenge and work with your extended network of suppliers and partners	120
Step 39	Automate processes to further improve quality and cost	122
Step 40	Learn from benchmark nonhealthcare organizations	122
Step 41	Learn from other benchmark healthcare organizations	127
Step 42	Learn from the institute for healthcare improvement	129
Step 43	Hold on to the gains you've achieved	129
Step 44	Reduce administrative overhead costs	130

Step 45   Avoid insurance company overhead costs   131
Step 46   Take a total systems view of healthcare for lean
improvement   132

**Chapter 4   A Capsule Summary of a Lean Toyota-like Production
System for Healthcare 135**

**Chapter 5   A Short To-Do List to Nationally Improve
U.S. Healthcare Cost and Quality 139**

Appendix A   Automaker Benchmarks   143

**Appendix B   Children's Hospital and Regional Medical
Center Emergency Department Patient Flow—Rapid
Process Improvement (RPI) 145**

**Appendix C   5-S Catches on at the VA Pittsburgh
Health System 151**

**Appendix D   Error-free Pathology: Applying Lean Production
Methods to Anatomic Pathology at the University of Pittsburgh
Shadyside Hospital 157**

Appendix E   Going Lean in Healthcare   191

Appendix F   Creating Lean Healthcare   213

Appendix G   Fixing Healthcare from the Inside, Today   229

Appendix H   Lean and Healthy   257

Appendix I   No Satisfaction at Toyota   267

Notes   279
Bibliography   285
Glossary of Lean Terms   289
Index   295

Preface

What differentiates this book from other healthcare improvement books is that it is the only currently available book that presents a simple recipe of 46 lean steps for healthcare providers to reduce cost and improve quality. By taking these straightforward steps, healthcare providers can adopt the same lean methods that have enabled companies like Toyota to become so successful.

This book has two teaching objectives. The reader will learn to:

1. Understand cost and quality issues facing healthcare in the United States.

2. Understand and implement a 46-step recipe to reduce healthcare costs and improve quality at healthcare providers by using Toyota lean production methods.

Although other books have presented Toyota's lean methods, this book goes further by showing how to directly apply those methods to healthcare, where they are sorely needed. This book is intended to be a practical manual for healthcare providers for improving quality and reducing costs. It represents a multiyear strategic direction for healthcare providers to adopt.

This second edition includes additional improvement steps and five new appendices of practical examples written by renowned lean experts. The author Robert Chalice may be contacted via email at authors@asq.org.

Acknowledgments

S pecial thanks go to the Institute for Healthcare Improvement (IHI) and all the authors of Appendix E "Going Lean in Healthcare": James Womack, PhD; Arthur Bryne, MBA; Orest Fiume, MA; Gary Kaplan, MD; and John Toussaint, MD. This is a remarkable group of experts who have made major contributions to lean healthcare.

Thank you also to George Alukal, for his co-authorship of Appendix F, "Creating Lean Healthcare." Mr. Alukal is a respected lean professional who is well known within the American Society for Quality.

Personal thanks go to Dr. Steven J. Spear of IHI and to Harvard Business Publishing for the excellent Appendix G, "Fixing Healthcare from the Inside, Today." Dr. Spear is a 2005 recipient of the Shingo prize for his paper, first published in the May 2004 issue of *Harvard Business Review*. The Shingo Prize, dubbed the "Nobel prize of Manufacturing" by *Business Week* in 2000, is a Utah State University award that recognizes contributions to business and manufacturing excellence.

Thank you to Andrew Scotchmer for Appendix H, "Lean and Healthy," which includes commentary on how lean is improving healthcare in Great Britain and the United States. This article first appeared in the August 2006 issue of *Qualityworld,* the magazine for the Institute of Quality Assurance (www.iqa.org/publication).

Thanks, also, to Charles Fishman for Appendix I, "No Satisfaction at Toyota," first published in *Fast Company* magazine, Issue 111, December 2006/January 2007.

Thank you to quality professional Barry Ross for his encouragement to add the change management and theory of constraints (that is, removing bottlenecks) improvement steps.

Many thanks go to Jennifer Condel, Anatomic Pathology Team leader; Dr. Stephen S. Raab, MD; David T. Sharbaugh; and Karen Wolk Feinstein, PhD at the University of Pittsburgh Medical Center Shadyside Hospital. They contributed an excellent lean case study in Appendix D, "Error-free Pathology: Applying Lean Production Methods to Anatomic Pathology." A related article, "Small Improvements Yield Big Results in Shadyside Pathology Lab," appears in the August 2004 newsletter of the Pittsburgh Regional Healthcare Initiative (PRHI) Web site, http://prhi.org/newsletters.cfm. The online article was written with the help of PRHI Communications Director Naida Grunden. The PRHI Web site, http://www.prhi.org, contains numerous improvement examples that may be replicated by other healthcare providers.

Thank you to communications director Naida Grunden, RN team leader Ellesha McCray, and CEO Michael Moreland for "5-S Catches On at the VA Pittsburgh Health System" in Appendix C.

Thank you to Barb Bouché, Continuous Performance Improvement manager at Seattle Children's Hospital and Regional Medical Center for the lean improvement example in Appendix B.

I wish to thank Lief Larson, CEO of Valhalla Worldwide LLC, for his review of the manuscript. I also wish to thank Mr. Dave LaCourse, IE, MS, for his past help, contributions, and encouragement. Thank you to Paul Spaude, past president of Aspirus Health System (Wausau, WI) and current president of Borgess Health Alliance (Kalamazoo, MI), for his review of an early manuscript.

Special thanks to Paul O'Mara, Matt Meinholz, and the folks at Thistle Hill Publishing Services for publishing assistance via the American Society for Quality.

Finally I wish to thank my stepmother and father, Eva and Walter, for their encouragement and guidance throughout my life, and my mother, Mae, for her nourishing love.

Part I

U.S. Healthcare System Problems and Solutions

1

U.S. Healthcare System Problems

RISING HEALTH INSURANCE PREMIUMS

Health coverage premiums rose at an annual rate of 7.7 percent in 2006, according to a survey of 3100 companies by the Kaiser Family Foundation done between January and May 2006.

A pessimistic cost outlook was released in November 2006 by PricewaterhouseCoopers, which reported that health benefit costs are expected to jump between 10.7 percent and 11.9 percent in 2007, depending on the insurance plan type. That increase would be more in line with the double-digit health benefit cost jumps during the 2001–2003 period that a Mercer report recalled. Thus Mercer is projecting that health insurance costs will continue increasing at double-digit rates.

Health insurance premiums have increased an average of 11 percent per year over the past 5 years (7.7 percent in 2006, 9.2 percent in 2005, 11.2 percent in 2004, 13.9 percent in 2003, and 12.9 percent in 2002). We are experiencing seemingly ever-increasing costs for health insurance. Over the past 7 years, health insurance premiums have approximately doubled. If the current trend continues, health coverage premiums will double again in about 7 years. By then, who will be able to afford it? Many companies with fewer than 25 employees have absorbed yearly premium increases of 25 percent or more. Imagine what you now pay for health coverage. Then imagine yourself paying double that in possibly less than 7 years. This crisis is happening now.

The graph in Figure 1.1 shows the year-to-year percentage change for health insurance premiums since 1988. The 2006 increase of 7.7 percent for health insurance premiums was approximately twice the general inflation rate of 3.5 percent, or the annual increase of worker earnings of about 3.8 percent. Over the last 20 years health insurance premiums have increased annually on average at approximately three times the annual inflation rate.

The graph in Figure 1.2 shows the corresponding annual premiums for employee-sponsored health insurance. The annual family health insurance premium grew to $11,480 in spring 2006, and the premiums for singles grew to $4,242 for employer-based coverage. In response, employers are shifting more and more healthcare costs to employees. Since 2000, the portion of the premium that employees pay has risen by nearly 50 percent. If you have the misfortune of paying for your own health coverage, you are in an ever-tightening vise of increasing costs. Check out your own health insurance premium increases this year—up by 12 percent, 22 percent, or possibly even 40 percent. My personal group health insurance premium went up by 33 percent in 2002, 10 percent in 2003, 29 percent in 2004, 14.5 percent in 2005, and 6.9 percent in 2006. My premiums

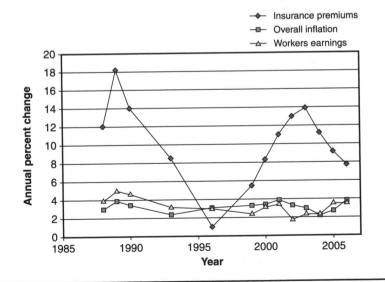

Figure 1.1   Year-to-year percentage change for health insurance premiums.

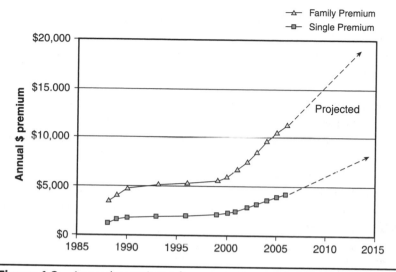

Figure 1.2 Annual premiums for employer-sponsored health insurance.

increased by 2.3 times in about 5 years and I'm not alone. So the problem we are now addressing in this book is "How do we stop these skyrocketing increases in healthcare costs?"[1]

Dr. W. Edwards Deming criticized "excessive medical costs" in the book *Four Days with Dr. Deming.*[2] Dr. Deming stated that his friend, William Hoglund, who was manager of Pontiac Motor Division prior to 1995, told him, "Blue Cross is our second largest supplier. The cost of medical care is $400 per car." Six months later Mr. Hoglund added that Blue Cross had overtaken steel as the most costly component in the automobile. That book was published over 10 years ago, and with sky-rocketing healthcare costs, the cost of healthcare in the automobile has risen from $400 then to $1500 now, that is, more than tripling. Relevant data from a GM source in 2006 are as follows:

- GM Spends $6 billion annually on healthcare.

- GM spends half as much on steel as it does on healthcare. Note that Starbucks also spends more on its healthcare than on coffee.

- Healthcare costs add about $1500 to the price of each GM car.

According to the United Autoworkers Union, "As of the second quarter of 2003, a UAW-represented assembler earns $25.63 per hour of straight time. A typical UAW-represented skilled-trades worker earns $29.75 per hour of straight time."[3] Appendix A shows that U.S. automobile manufacturers generally expend about 25 labor hours per manufactured vehicle. So if we use a worker's wage of $30 per hour times 25 hours per vehicle, the cost of labor in each vehicle is about $750. Therefore, GM's current cost for healthcare of $1500 per vehicle is also almost double its labor cost of $750 per vehicle. The healthcare cost per vehicle is now greater than either the cost of the steel or the workers' wages in each manufactured vehicle.

On February 11, 2005, the *Washington Post* published an article titled "U.S. Firms Losing Health Care Battle, GM Chairman Says." Statements from that article include:

> American manufacturers are losing their ability to compete in the global marketplace in large measure because of the crushing burden of health care costs, General Motors Corp. chairman and chief executive G. Richard Wagoner Jr. said as he called on corporate and government leaders to find "some serious medicine" for the nation's ailing health system.
>
> In a speech at the Economic Club of Chicago, the auto executive, who is responsible for providing health insurance for more people than any other private employer in the nation, graphically detailed how rising medical bills are eating into his company's bottom line and ultimately threatening the viability of most U.S. firms.
>
> "Failing to address the health care crisis would be the worst kind of procrastination," Wagoner said, "the kind that places our children and our grandchildren at risk and threatens the health and global competitiveness of our nation's economy.
>
> "GM and the United Auto Workers didn't cause this double-digit inflation in health care," he said. And if GM pushed for sharp reductions in health benefits, the powerful union would likely strike and send the company into Chapter 11 bankruptcy protection, he predicted.
>
> But the figure that prompted Wagoner to raise his voice is $1,500. That is the amount of money added to the price of

every single vehicle to cover health care, a cost that his foreign competitors do not bear.

"The cost of health care in the U.S. is making American businesses extremely uncompetitive versus our global counterparts," he said. "In the U.S., health care costs have been rising at double-digit rates for many years.

"That huge benefit hit is chewing up the salaries and wages we would be receiving," he said. "That's the key."

Wagoner broke his silence on some type of national catastrophic reinsurance program or using a separate government-backed insurance pool to cover the most expensive medical cases.

"If we can create a comprehensive insurance model to better share these catastrophic costs among all consumers, then we can take a big step toward providing affordable health care coverage for all our citizens," Wagoner said.

"It's simply not acceptable for over 46 million Americans to be without health care coverage. And it's unfair for those of us who do provide health care benefits to have to pay higher bills to cover the costs of the uninsured."

The business leaders cannot understand why the health care industry has been slow to institute the sort of technological changes that helped them improve quality and reduce costs.

"Only in health care does bad service and bad quality get paid for in the same manner as good service and good quality," said Humana Inc. chief executive Michael B. McCallister, chairman of the Business Roundtable's health care task force.

The CEOs agree that the double-digit premium increases will continue as long as individuals are sheltered from the true cost of health care.

In November 2006, the CEOs of GM, Ford, and Chrysler met with President George W. Bush to discuss the spiraling healthcare costs manufacturers face. GM is the largest private purchaser of healthcare in the United States. A GM spokesman stated that while the company understands that they have to "win," there are issues like healthcare that affect competitive balance. In fact all three automakers spend more on healthcare per vehicle than on steel;

healthcare adds $1000 to $1500 per car for each of them. The CEO of GM also urged Congress to provide a "vigorous and robust" prescription drug market.

Consider again that automobile manufacturers now expend only about 25 hours of labor per each vehicle manufactured. That's rather astounding! These manufacturers can now make an entire automobile with just 25 hours of assembly workers' labor. That's because they have been continuously improving their processes, quality, and costs for years. Because of intense foreign competition, they must either improve or disappear. Healthcare can similarly follow their example to improve.

It is becoming increasingly difficult for American manufacturers to compete in world markets because of continually rising healthcare costs. Similarly, school and city budgets have been hard hit by annual health insurance increases. Teacher counts and city services are being reduced to compensate for premium increases. For that matter, every purchaser of healthcare has been adversely affected.

The graph shown in Figure 1.3 illustrates changes in healthcare costs compared to other components of the consumer price index (CPI) between 1990 and 2005. What we see is that the cost of hospital services, nursing home, and adult day care increased 2.7-fold from 1990 to 2005. If hospital services costs were presented alone without nursing homes and adult day care, the increase would probably have been much greater, possibly the highest on the graph. It is little comfort to see that only college tuition and natural gas costs have had a greater increase. Also note that prescription drugs and medical supply costs increased 2.1-fold, while physician service costs increased 1.9-fold from 1990 to 2005. You usually hear people complain about continuing cost increases for cable TV, natural gas, gasoline, and electricity, but the fact is that hospital and other healthcare costs have outpaced them by a wide margin. Something has to be done to slow the steady rise of healthcare costs—*that something is improving healthcare processes using the lean production methods described in this book.* One consolation from the chart is that televisions and personal computers now cost you about half than they did in 1990. Unfortunately the costs for episodes of individual healthcare are also far greater in magnitude than most items on the chart. A hospital discharge might cost you more than $15,000 (not

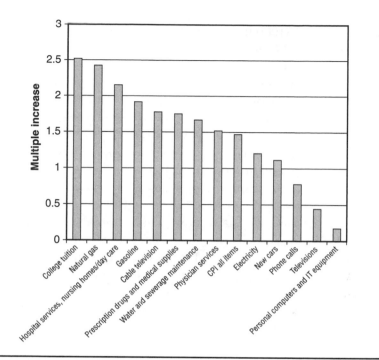

Figure 1.3 Price in 2005 / price in 1990.

counting doctors' charges) and it's increasing steadily. That's a lot more than a tank of gas or a monthly cable TV or home heating bill.[4]

WHY DOUBLE-DIGIT HEALTH INSURANCE INCREASES?

Why does the cost of health insurance coverage continue to increase at double-digit rates? Could it be that hospitals (and possibly physicians) generally represent near monopolies in their service areas? If you're having a heart attack, are you going to question the cost of care at the nearest hospital? Insured patients (governmental and commercially insured) make up 84 percent of the U.S. population and usually don't question healthcare charges even if they are exorbitant, because their insurance will pay most of it. Insurance softens the blow of excessive costs, even if insurance premiums continually go up. How often do patients with insurance ask for the price of procedures prior to care? Not very often, because someone else is paying the bill. If each person were spending only their own hard-earned dollars, there would be far more scrutiny.

Table 1.1 is from Lucette Lagnado's article "California Hospitals Open Books, Showing Huge Price Differences."[5]

A law enacted in California in 2004 requires hospitals to disclose the list prices of each patient chargeable item. Prior to this law, California hospitals, like nearly all other hospitals in the United States, kept their price lists secret. Patients generally had no idea of the gamut of charges they would face until they received their final bill. The new California law, as well as initiatives in a few other states like Arizona, Wisconsin, and Minnesota, is, thankfully, beginning to change this situation. What is surprising is that these disclosures show that prices can vary as much as 17-fold from one hospital to the next for the same item or service. Table 1.1 shows, for example, that a "CT-scan of the head without contrast" varies from a low of $881 to a high of $4,037, a rather remarkable difference. What's bothersome is that these kinds of price variations are common when comparing random hospitals across the United States. This is a problem for consumers as well as the health care industry to address.

Table 1.1   How much is that chest x-ray?

A new California law allows patients to look up the retail prices of many goods and services at hospitals. A survey of several hospital price lists shows dramatic differences in price.

	Scripps Memorial La Jolla, San Diego	Sutter General, Sacramento	UC Davis, Sacramento	San Francisco General, San Francisco	Doctors, Modesto	Cedars-Sinai Los Angeles	West Hills Hospital, West Hills
Chest X-ray (two views, basic)	$120.90	$790	$451.50	$120	$1,519	$412.90	$396.77
Complete blood count	$47	$234	$166	$50	$547.30	$165.80	$172.42
Comprehensive metabolic panel	$196.60	$743	$451**	$97	$1,732.95	$576	$387.18
CT-scan, head/brain (without contrast)	$881.90	$2,807	$2,868	$950	$6,599	$4,037.61	$2,474.95
Percocet* (or Crycodone hydrochloride and acetaminophen) one tablet, 5–325 mg	$11.44	$26.79	$15	$6.68	$35.50	$6.50	$27.86
Tylenol* (or acetaminophen) one tablet, 325 mg	$7.06	No charge	$1	$5.50	No charge	12 cents	$3.28

* Hospitals carry either generic version, name brand, or both
** Represents the added total of 14 tests that make up the comprehensive metabolic panel
Sources: Scripps Memorial, La Jolla; Sutter General; UC Davis Health System; San Francisco General; Doctors Medical Center; Cedars-Sinai Health System; West Hills Hospital and Medical Center

Some semblance of rational pricing needs to prevail here. Admittedly, many patients do not pay list prices because they are part of an HMO or insurance group that has negotiated better pricing, or they are Medicare patients for whom the government pays a fixed amount based on their diagnosis and care episode. Unfortunately, the patients who are billed list prices are generally those without insurance and who are the least able to pay since they have the least market clout. Lucette Lagnado's *Wall Street Journal* article states, "The elaborate pricing systems hospitals have developed over the years will be difficult to change, many in the industry say." Jan Emerson, spokeswoman for the California Healthcare Association, adds, "The entire system will have to be blown up." Clearly reform is needed here.

Care for Ohio, an organization sponsored by a healthcare union, states, "If you have no health insurance or your health insurance doesn't cover your bill, chances are you'll be expected to pay more than twice the price insured patients pay for the same treatment. Care for Ohio is a project launched by the members of SEIU District 1199, Ohio's healthcare union, to shine a light on the practices of hospitals. The organization makes information available to patients, consumers, hospital employees, taxpayers, elected leaders, and community advocates to help promote the best decisions about health care—and it makes sure hospitals do their share to care for Ohio. In March 2005, Care for Ohio published an outstanding report titled "Twice the Price—What Uninsured and Under Insured Patients Pay for Hospital Care." It states, "If health insurance doesn't cover your bill, you're in for a severe case of sticker shock." A billing system that charges twice as much to those who can least afford healthcare is clearly broken.[6]

Care for Ohio recommends:

> The ultimate solution, of course, is to create a health care system that guarantees everyone access to affordable health care. In the meantime, there are steps Ohio (and other states) can take to stop the overcharging of the uninsured, including: 1) Set limits on the prices hospitals can charge uninsured and underinsured patients, so that they will not be required to pay more for necessary medical care than it costs hospitals to provide it. 2) Create uniform charity care standards

defining the amount of free and discounted care hospitals are expected to provide patients in need. 3) Require far greater transparency and disclosure so that Ohio (and other) hospitals make their prices more accessible to consumers, publicize the availability of charity care, and report to the state annually the number and income of self-paying patients, the prices charged and free care provided, and the actual cost of providing the care.

Although Care for Ohio's recommendations are important, they do not reduce the fundamental existing waste and inefficiency in related healthcare processes. It's important to go beyond the recommendations to improve the care delivery processes by eliminating all forms of waste.

When there is more than one healthcare provider in a service area, how much duplicate technology and facility are there and how much does that add to the overall cost of healthcare? As an example, former U.S. Senator David Durenberger of Minnesota noted in a 2005 presentation that there are 21 CT scanners within 2.1 miles of Fairview Southdale Hospital near Minneapolis. Is that rational from a cost perspective, or does it reflect a healthcare system that is simply out of control?

Healthcare providers operate, by their own nature, in a "survival mode." Each is trying to overcome the others in a race for market share, growth, and dominance. Competing providers do not generally operate in a synergistic manner to complement one another. Their goal is to simply capture and maintain market share. Shouldn't their goal instead be to achieve the best health care status at the lowest cost for the entire population of a region? For years (see Figure 1.1) healthcare providers have chosen to increase costs rather than embrace lean delivery methods to lower costs, or even keep costs the same from year to year. At the same time, providers continually try to increase prices and profits to the extent that employers and the public will endure. Some healthcare administrators have told me they are concerned that reducing costs may cause patients to perceive they are receiving lower quality. It makes one wonder what will indeed motivate hospital administrators to lower costs. They don't seem to wish to do it voluntarily. If a healthcare provider embraced lean methods to lower cost, it would force competing providers to eventually follow suit. According to the Wisconsin Hospital Association (WHA), the reasons for escalating costs include:

1. Advances in patient care—Advances in medical treatments and technologies mean higher survival rates and safer, more convenient hospital services. Some prescription drugs for example are astronomically expensive. These advances are costly to fund.

2. Input costs—Workforce shortages are driving up healthcare worker salaries at rates much higher than inflation.

3. Government underfunding—The Medicare and Medicaid programs dramatically underpay their fair share of hospital expenses, forcing hospitals to shift costs to private payers.

4. Employer-sponsored health insurance—Lack of economic consequences for employees leads to higher consumption.

5. Less than optimum care—The Midwest Business Group on Health (MBGH) says 30 percent of cost of care is due to poor quality.

46.6 MILLION AMERICANS (ALMOST 1 IN 6) ARE WITHOUT HEALTH INSURANCE

In 2005, the number of Americans without health insurance rose by 1.3 million to 46.6 million, or 15.9 percent of the population.[7] That's more than the combined population of the nation's 24 least populous states plus the District of Columbia. It's also about 1.25 times the entire population of the most populous state, California. Imagine all the people in California representing far less than the total uninsured in the United States.

Figure 1.4 is a remarkable graph of the U.S. trend in uninsured from the Commonwealth Fund. It is not that far off until one in five Americans will lack health insurance. It is a sad commentary that the United States, one of the richest nations in the world, is yet incapable of guaranteeing basic healthcare for its citizens.

In August 2006, the U.S. Census Bureau released figures showing that 15.9 percent of Americans were uninsured during 2005, compared

Number of uninsured, in millions

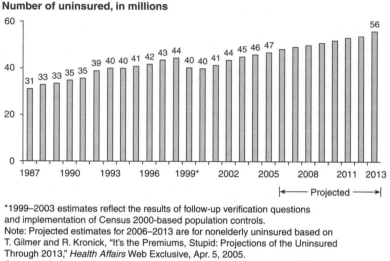

*1999–2003 estimates reflect the results of follow-up verification questions and implementation of Census 2000-based population controls.
Note: Projected estimates for 2006–2013 are for nonelderly uninsured based on T. Gilmer and R. Kronick, "It's the Premiums, Stupid: Projections of the Uninsured Through 2013," *Health Affairs* Web Exclusive, Apr. 5, 2005.
Source: U.S. Census Bureau, March CPS Surveys 1988 to 2005.

Figure 1.4   47 million uninsured in 2005; increasing steadily since 2000.

Source: Commonwealth Fund, 1 East 75th Street, New York, NY 10021. Phone: 212.606.3800 Fax: 212.606.3500. http://www.cmwf.org.

to 15.6 percent in 2004, 15.5 percent in 2003, 15.2 percent in 2002, and 14.6 percent in 2001. This increasing trend in the number of uninsured is ominous. In 2003, there was an increase of 1.5 million uninsured compared to a 2.4 million increase in 2002. The total increase of 3.9 million uninsured in 2002 and 2003 is larger than the population of either metropolitan Los Angeles or Chicago, which are the second and third largest cities in the United States, exceeded only by the population of metropolitan New York. Understand that the group of uninsured in the United States actually grew during 2002 and 2003 by an amount larger than metropolitan Los Angeles' population! Nearly one in six U.S. citizens did not have health insurance coverage during 2005. One in four residents of New Mexico and Texas presently lacks health insurance. There are more than 8 million uninsured children in the United States. The rising cost of healthcare coverage is contributing to the growing crisis of the uninsured. In 2005 the percentage of people covered by employer-based health insurance fell to 59.5 percent, compared to 59.8 percent in 2004, 60.4 percent in 2003, and 61.3 percent in 2002, no doubt due to increasing cost.

In the United States it is a right of each citizen to receive a public education through high school. Should it not also be a right of each U.S. citizen to receive affordable health insurance and affordable healthcare? The CEO of a large U.S. healthcare system once commented to me that when he looked at the list of personal bankruptcies frequently published in the local newspaper, he observed that the majority was due to healthcare-related bills. In 2005, a Harvard study concluded that half of all U.S. bankruptcies filers stated that medical expenses led to their financial downfall and most of them had health insurance.[8] They also found a 30-fold increase in medically related bankruptcies compared to a similar study conducted in 1981. Medical bankruptcies affect up to 2.2 million Americans.[9] Isn't it time that we as a nation provide our citizens with a basic level of healthcare so that major illnesses don't leave them destitute?

MOTIVATING HEALTHCARE PROVIDERS TO REDUCE COST AND IMPROVE QUALITY

An important question is what will motivate healthcare providers, particularly hospitals, to truly embrace high-quality, lean production methods? As long as patients and employers continue to accept and endure continually rising healthcare premiums and costs, there is little hope. When the cost of healthcare becomes so outrageous that individuals and employers can no longer afford it, then change may occur as they clamor. After the cost of healthcare doubles again, picket lines may appear in front of healthcare facilities and insurers. This may come to pass within the next seven years, as healthcare costs are projected to double again. A few scenarios are possible: (1) Public and employer outrage will produce meaningful voluntary cost reduction; (2) Partial government intervention (and cost control) will occur; (3) the U.S. healthcare system will be nationalized, as it is in many other countries, such as Canada; or (4) the U.S. may adopt a hybrid system, as in France, that guarantees basic benefits and allows citizens to purchase more comprehensive insurance benefits. While some may argue against nationalized healthcare in the United States, nearly everyone agrees that U.S. healthcare has simply become too expensive. Healthcare providers and insurers have not held down or reduced costs on their own. Healthcare costs are presently rising at about five times the rate of overall inflation (see Figure 1.1). Few if any would disagree with the objective of simply reducing U.S. healthcare costs.

One may ask why healthcare providers have not yet embraced lean methods as other U.S. manufacturers have. To be frank, many healthcare providers are near monopolies in their service areas. They have had little reason to embrace lean. By comparison, a manufacturer with increasingly low cost foreign competition from China, Asia, or Mexico has been forced to embrace lean or face extinction.

Healthcare worker shortages may encourage providers to embrace lean methods to be more efficient with limited available talent. From 2004 to 2014, employment in healthcare occupations is expected to grow 26 percent, or twice the 13 percent growth rate of nonhealthcare jobs. During that 10-year period, job growth of between 34 percent and 56 percent is expected for personal care aides, medical assistants, and physician assistants, medical record technicians, home health aides, physical and occupational therapy aides and assistants, and audiologists.[10]

A 2004 report, "Manufacturing in America—A Comprehensive Strategy to Address the Challenges to U.S. Manufacturers" by the U.S. Department of Commerce—lists *reducing healthcare costs as the number one priority.*[11] Between 2000 and 2003, the U.S. lost 15.1 percent, or 2.6 million, of its manufacturing jobs. The report states, "The challenges confronting American manufacturers and manufacturing workers are urgent, and President Bush has already taken action. He has implemented a jobs and growth agenda and outlined a six-point plan." Note the number one priority is to reduce healthcare costs.

1. To make healthcare costs more affordable

2. To reduce the lawsuit burden on the U.S. economy

3. To ensure an affordable, reliable energy supply

4. To streamline regulations and reporting requirements

5. To open markets for American products

6. To enable families and businesses to plan for the future with confidence

A typical U.S. small/medium manufacturer would sum up the healthcare cost problem as follows:

> Healthcare is a big concern that we have in keeping competitive. We spend about $9000 per employee on healthcare, and when half of our people make under $30,000 a year, it is hard to make ends meet. The rising cost of healthcare is the biggest barrier to health coverage. The annual family health insurance premium grew to $11,480 in spring 2006 while insurance premiums for singles grew to $4242 for employer-based coverage. Note that the family healthcare premium is more than one third of the employee's salary. In 2007, it cost nearly $7 per hour to pay for a small business employee's family health insurance premium. Some have projected that by 2010, the cost of healthcare for small business will be more than the employee wages themselves. Insurance premiums for small business have been growing fastest. What these facts suggest is that there is competitive value for reducing healthcare costs that U.S. manufacturing companies face, particularly for small and medium-sized manufacturers that are the foundation of the U.S. manufacturing sector.

What's in it for hospital administrators to embrace lean? (WIFM = "What's in It for Me?") To date they haven't done so voluntarily. The following points may encourage some administrators to embrace lean. This is a pivotal point. If there isn't enough incentive to promote positive change, healthcare leaders and their organizations will adhere to the status quo of increasing costs and ok-marginal quality. Healthcare leaders may not be experiencing the kind of "burning platform" that forced most U.S. manufacturers to embrace lean to simply survive against growing Chinese, Mexican, and Asian competition. If hospital administrators would embrace a lean system, they would:

- Produce meaningful cost and quality improvement
- Achieve strategic advantage over competition
- Quell growing business and public clamoring about healthcare costs
- Earn greater prestige—national recognition
- Generate greater profit

- Provide funds for uninsured, uncompensated care, and philanthropy

- Help fend off government intervention, cost control, and nationalized healthcare

- Better use increasingly scarce healthcare workers

TOYOTA LEAN PRODUCTION

To solve the problems of rising healthcare costs and questionable quality, we will turn to the techniques used by one of the most successful automobile companies in the world, the Toyota Motor Company. On May 3, 2003, the *Detroit News* published an article headlined "Profit-Rich Toyota Threatens Big Three—Can Anything Stop Toyota?" An article on May 11, 2006, exclaimed, "Toyota Profits Jump to $12 Billion" for its fiscal year ending that March. That was nearly double GM's peak annual earnings of $6.9 billion in 1995. It is also more than any Detroit automaker has made in any one year since at least the 1960s and more than GM, Ford, and Chrysler made combined in any recent year. These companies have faced hardships while Japan-based Toyota is enjoying soaring profits.

In the fiscal year ending January 31, 2006, Toyota continued to grow its net profits by a stunning 17 percent. Toyota moved in front of Ford in 2004 to become the world's second largest automobile producer, behind only GM. Based on the current trend, Toyota will overtake GM as the world's largest car company by 2010 with a 15 percent worldwide market share. This is an ominous sign for U.S. automobile manufacturing. By implementing what has become know as the "Toyota Lean Production System (TPS)," Toyota has become the de facto standard of performance for companies. Health care providers can similarly adopt some of Toyota's successful methods to reduce cost and improve quality.

By contrast, the U.S. automakers are struggling. GM lost $3.4 billion in the quarter ending June 2006. Ford reported its largest-ever annual loss of $12.7 billion in 2006. This amounts to a loss of $4380 on each car or truck they sold in 2006. Ford's annual sales dropped about 10 percent that year. GM and Ford shares traded at lows not seen in more than a decade. GM has cited rising medical costs as contributing to its losses. It said that U.S. healthcare costs continue to grow at an excessive rate, which hampers profitability. It will spend $6 billion in 2006 on health insurance to cover over a million salaried and hourly workers, retirees, and family members. Moody's Investors Service and Fitch Ratings cut GM's debt rating to one notch above junk status. Ford Motor and DaimlerChrysler are similarly hurt by rising healthcare costs.

GM and Ford are both engaged in large downsizing plans. GM has persuaded about 35,000 hourly workers to leave the company under early retirement or buyout plans, and Ford has offered buyouts and early retirement packages to all 75,000 U.S. production workers. Ford hopes to reduce its hourly workforce by as many as 30,000 and is expected to shutter 16 plants.

On October 4, 2006, a small piece on Bloomberg.com stated: "Toyota takes off. Toyota Motor Corp. hammered its U.S. rivals again last month. Toyota's U.S. sales soared by 25 percent over a year earlier; General Motors and Chrysler's domestic sales slipped, and Ford saw a 4.7 percent increase." David Hilton of Cap Gemini added, "It doesn't look like anything can stop Toyota, or even slow them down." Then on October 13 the news was, "Big Japanese automakers made $2,400 more than their U.S. rivals on every car they sold in North America last year. They accomplished the feat by charging more, and spending less on labor and health care."

Realize that Toyota was nearly bankrupt in 1949 and terminated a large part of its workforce. By implementing what has become known as the Toyota Lean Production System (TPS), Toyota has become the benchmark by which American automobile executives judge their own companies. Compared to traditional mass production techniques, Toyota manufactures with half the human effort in the factory, half the manufacturing space, half the investment tools, half the engineering hours, and half the time to develop new products. Despite being the most efficient carmaker in the world, Toyota produces world-class-quality automobiles.

In the August 2006 J. D. Powers Dependability Study, Toyota models dominated their segment rankings. Toyota captured the best dependability rankings with four models. Toyota also had the highest customer retention rate in the automobile industry. That is, a higher percentage of Toyota owners repurchase another Toyota, as compared to any other automobile brand.

Similarly, the April 2005 *Consumer Reports* Reliability Study ranked 10 Japanese models "most reliable," and there were no U.S. domestic models in the top 10. The April 2005 *Consumer Reports* "Quick Picks" of "82 best cars" based on high ratings, reliability, fuel economy, safety, and overall satisfaction included no domestic models. This issue had a list of 32 cars that more than 80 percent of consumers would "purchase again." That list contained 25 Japanese models, dominated by Toyota, and only one U.S. model, the Chevrolet Corvette.

In the March 2006 *Consumer Reports* Reliability Study, Japanese automakers were again the best and most reliable. Asian vehicles took all the spots in the "top picks" list for the first time ever. The results are a setback for Ford and General Motors.

Of the 69 cars and trucks *Consumer Reports* rated "good bets" for used-car buyers, 59 carried Japanese nameplates, while just 8 were from domestic brands. American brands accounted for 22 of the 34 "bad bets"—a list that included no Japanese models. *Consumer Reports,* published by the nonprofit Consumers Union, bases its top picks on the findings of a team of engineers and technicians who test vehicles and on its survey results.

The Toyota Lean Production System is what Toyota uses to deliver best quality, lowest cost, and shortest product manufacturing time though the incessant elimination of waste. Toyota focuses on the tasks and responsibilities of those workers, who actually add value to the car, and reduces or eliminates all other non-value-added tasks and labor. TPS is composed of three pillars: just-in-time production with just-in-time inventory; built-in quality at each step without the need for reinspection; and respect for the employee. *Quality* is defined as "meeting or exceeding customer expectations." Alternatively it may be defined as "meeting or exceeded predefined standards." Either definition is workable and interchangeable. Clearly, American industry and by extension the U.S. healthcare system has much to learn from Toyota's efficient yet high-quality methods.

The Lean Enterprise Institute defines *lean production* as follows:

> A business system for organizing and managing product (or service) development, operations, suppliers, and customer (patient) relations that requires less human effort, less space, less capital, and less time to make products (services) with fewer defects to precise customer desires, compared with the previous system.[12]

Lean production was pioneered by Toyota after World War II and, as of 1990, typically required half the human effort, half the manufacturing space and capital investment for a given amount of capacity, and a fraction of the development and lead time of mass production systems, while making products in wider variety at lower volumes with many fewer defects. The term was coined by John Krafcik, a research assistant at MIT with the International Motor Vehicle Program in the late 1980s.

Lean thinking is a five-step thought process proposed by James Womack and Dan Jones in their 1996 book *Lean Thinking* to guide managers through a lean transformation.[13] The steps are:

1. Specify value from the standpoint of the end customer

2. Identify all the steps in the value stream

3. Make the value creating steps flow toward the customer

4. Let customers pull value (toward them) from the next upstream activity

5. Pursue perfection

WASTE IN HEALTHCARE

Don Berwick, MD president and CEO of the Institute for Healthcare Improvement (IHI), estimates that 30 to 40 percent of the total cost of healthcare production is waste or, as the Japanese call it, *muda*. Cindy Jimmerson, a nurse who has also been pursuing lean health-care methods states, "The national numbers for waste in healthcare are between 30 percent and 40 percent, but the reality of what we've observed doing minute-by-minute observation over the last three years is closer to 60 percent. That's waste of time, waste of money, waste of material resources. It's nasty. The waste is not limited to administrative costs, which most research on health-care has documented. It's everywhere: patient care and non-patient care alike." Jim Womack, PhD., founder of the Lean Enterprise Institute, similarly estimates that organizations can generally save 50 percent of labor and space by converting to lean production methods similar to Toyota's. Is it possible that our healthcare delivery system can similarly save 50 percent by converting to lean production? By *lean production,* we mean the elimination of waste in all its forms whether time, materials, or unneeded process steps. By *lean processes,* we don't mean making employees work harder. We do mean eliminating all waste and non-value-added steps in work processes to improve cost and quality. The healthcare industry itself has much to gain by adopting Toyota's lean methods, as I will further present. What is most critical for U.S. healthcare executives is to embed into their organizations a mind-set of continuous cost and quality improvement. This means setting a goal that there will be no cost (or insurance premium) increase this year for our patients. Even better, there will be an X percent cost reduction, and we will simultaneously achieve quality improvement goals and specific community health objectives.

Cost per case mix indexed (CMI) adjusted patient discharge is defined as the cost per discharged patient adjusted for patient severity. It is a comparable cost indicator across all hospitals. Why is there such huge variability in cost per CMI adjusted discharge across the country from around $5000 at the lowest-cost hospitals to more than $15,000 per discharge at the highest-cost hospitals? You may pay a different price for the same hospital stay or medical procedure all across the country. There is little consistency in the actual price and quality of medical care across the United States.

EXCESS HEALTHCARE ADMINISTRATIVE AND OVERHEAD COSTS

Many health care CEO salaries in 2003 ranged from $600,000 up to $2 million and are likely much higher today.[14] One CEO earned about $2.34 million per year in 2003, or about $1125 per hour. That CEO's salary appears to have increased about 62 percent from 2002 to 2003. Ask any one of the 46 million uninsured in the United States, or any small employer who has just had a 30 percent health insurance premium increase, whether such hospital administrator salaries seem reasonable. A $2.34 million salary equates to the combined salary of about 45 RNs capable of simultaneously caring for about 270 med/surg patients. Can these kinds of administrative dollars be better spent? What's of more value—one administrator or 45 nurses delivering patient care?

With 1 in 6 people in the U.S being uninsured, is it rational for any nonprofit health system board to approve a CEO's salary of $2.34 million per year knowing that many uninsured patients will be helping pay it?

Executives at the six largest nonprofit, tax-exempt hospital systems all make more than $1.2 million a year. One large system has given $5.1 million in forgivable loans to eight top executives since 1998. Another paid $185,427 in 2005 so two executives could live in other states and commute to work.[15] In a Catholic not-for-profit healthcare system, a CEO's salary was about $1 million in 2001 and was increased by $640,000 or 64 percent within the following 3 years. Do RNs or other frontline healthcare workers ever receive such a percentage salary increase?

Some individual annual salaries for CEOs at 300- to 500-bed community hospitals commonly reach $500,000 and beyond. Look within your own community. If your local hospital has more than 300 beds, you'll probably find that its hospital administrator is making more than your mayor, your superintendent of schools, your governor, most local corporate executives, and even the president of the United States. By the way, the salary of the president of the United States is $400,000 per year.

By contrast, there are some good examples of rational CEO salaries in U.S. companies. For example, the CEO of the discount retailer Costco had a salary of $350,000 in 2006. Costco had 2006 annual revenue of about $62 billion. It is a large and profitable company. Yet its CEO receives a more reasonable annual salary than many healthcare CEOs. It is true that Costco's CEO receives stock options, which are a type of bonus that appreciates based on the performance of the company's stock. Still, Costco represents a good example of rational CEO compensation in business that healthcare organizations may emulate.

Table 1.2 shows that in 2003 hospital presidents and CEOs in Ontario, Canada, earned an average of $239,000—that's in Canadian dollars (CAD), which equals approximately $210,000 in U.S. dollars (USD). So, it appears that in 2003 the Canadian Universal Healthcare System rewarded the average hospital CEO a salary of $210,000 USD, which is about 47 percent less than his average U.S. counterpart earning approximately $390,000 USD per year. So to some extent, the Canadian Healthcare System contains healthcare costs by containing administrative salaries.

Table 1.2   Ontario 2003 healthcare executive salaries.
($1 Canadian = approximately $0.88 USD)

Occupation	Average Income 2003	Average Income Annual Growth 1996–2003	Number of Employees Annual Growth 1996–2003	Total Income 2003 $M
Executives	$208,344	3.8%	8.9%	$63
President & CEO	$239,327	5.4%	4.7%	$28
Medical executives	$198,361	2.0%	6.9%	$14
Other nonmedical executives	$182,674	4.6%	17.6%	$20
Nonexecutives	$148,620	1.5%	18.0%	$247
All earners over $100,000	$157,762	1.7%	16.2%	$309

Source: Government of Ontario, http://www.fraserinstitute.ca/admin/books/files/
WhereTheMoneyGoes.pdf

In 2003, it was also true that a hospital CEO in Ontario with an average annual salary of about $239,000 CAD earned approximately 4.6 times a Canadian RN's salary of about $52,000 CAD. Maybe the U.S. healthcare system can learn from the Canadian system by adopting a guideline that a U.S. hospital CEO or administrator's salary should not exceed 5 times the average registered nurse's salary. Or should Congress consider a law to that effect? In reality some U.S. hospital executives earn more than 50 to 100 times the average registered nurse's salary. Even limiting U.S. healthcare executive compensation to 10 times the average RN salary would be a vast improvement compared to present excesses.

What is a logical way for a hospital board to reward a CEO consistent with a lean philosophy? First, set the base pay at reasonable level of approximately five times the average RN's salary. Then provide the CEO with a bonus up to 30 percent of salary based on simultaneously achieving patient satisfaction, employee satisfaction, physician satisfaction, quality, cost, and earnings goals. Annual goals would be continuously improved from year to year. Rewarding CEOs at healthcare providers in such a manner would be a win-win for all.

Realize also that each RN simultaneously cares for approximately six patients on a general med/surg hospital unit. This means that 10 RNs may care for as many as 60 patients simultaneously. Should any healthcare executive be paid more than 10 RNs able to care for 60 patients simultaneously? Hospital boards should each ask themselves that precise question. How are salary dollars best spent to provide true value added services to patients? If executive salaries were more reasonable, there would still be no shortage of well-qualified applicants for these high-paying jobs. Linking hospital CEO salaries to a multiple of RN salaries like 5 to 10 would also make it less likely for CEOs to reduce RN direct-care salaries, since that would in effect reduce their own salaries. It would encourage CEOs to instead remove other sources of waste, focus on providing even more direct patient care, and even increase RN salaries.

Note that the average salary of a registered nurse in the U.S. is also about $52,000 USD per year, which is about 12 percent more than the similar $52,000 CAD average Canadian RN salary. So it appears that the Canadian Health System is also containing nursing costs.

Consider Figure 1.5, which shows the growth of hospital administrative personnel compared to the growth in RN caregivers.[16] Wouldn't it make more sense to instead increase the growth in RNs? Note that physician growth versus administrator growth chart is very similar.

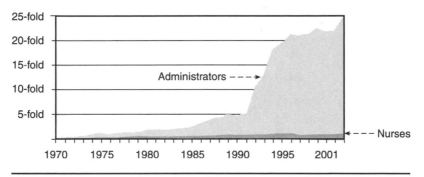

Figure 1.5 Increases in registered nurses versus administrators.
Source: Bureau of Labor Statistics and Center for Policy Studies.

EXCESS INSURANCE COMPANY ADMINISTRATIVE AND OVERHEAD COSTS

In reality, health insurance companies are adding approximately 20 percent to 30 percent overhead to patient care costs, or about 10 times the overhead that Medicare adds.

Figure 1.6 shows some sample overhead percentages.

Excess insurance company overhead is due to inflated executive salaries, profits, buildings, and capital expenditures. Should Congress consider a law that all health management and health insurance companies can add no more than 10 percent overhead to the actual cost of patient care? That compares to only 3 percent overhead that the Medicare system currently adds. That would contain their profits and operating costs, including their CEO salaries and capital costs, such as buildings. In fact, Governor Arnold Schwarzenegger's 2007 California Plan for Healthcare would limit insurance company overhead to about 15 percent of premiums and cover all California residents.[17] Or, somehow, the United States might simply reduce reliance on health insurance companies, as Maine and Massachusetts seem to be doing.

As you can see from Table 1.3, it is not uncommon for health management or health insurance company CEO's to earn salaries of $10 million or more per year, besides owning company shares if publicly traded. Of particular note on the following list is the past CEO of United Healthcare, who earned about $10 million in 2005

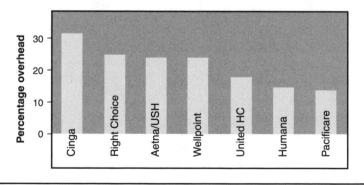

Figure 1.6   Health insurance company overhead.

Source: BestWeek Life/special Rep 4/12/1999.

Table 1.3 2005 CEO compensation at selected health management and insurance companies.

Company	Pay (millions of dollars)	Five-year Pay (millions of dollars)	Shares Owned (millions of dollars)	Age
Caremark Rx	69.66	161.85	3.9	57
Aetna	30.86‡	N/A	32.5	57
Cigna	28.82	78.31	79.7	54
United Health Group	10.70	297.21	36.6	58
WellPoint	10.16†	56.95	34.8	58
Coventry Health Care	7.46††	N/A	14.0	50
Omnicare	6.02†	39.78	121.9	66
HCA	3.74†	14.30	15.2	60
Tenet Healthcare	3.64	9.70*	2.8	46
Humana	3.33	15.10	18.6	53
Health Management	1.71	17.37	13.5	60

Methodology: Total 2005 compensation for each chief executive includes the following: salary and bonuses; other compensation, such as vested restricted stock grants, Long-Term Incentive Plan (LTIP) payouts and perks; and stock gains, the value realized by exercising stock options.

*Three-year total.
†Prior-year data.
‡New chief executive; compensation may be for another executive officer.

Sources: http://www.forbes.com, "Top Earning CEOs' list", latest company proxy statements; FT Interactive Data via FactSet Research Systems; Hemscott, Inc., http://www.hemscottdata.com.

and about $297 million over five years (that is, nearly $60 million per year). He accumulated a net worth of nearly a billion dollars as CEO with United Healthcare, a Minnesota health insurance company. That's billion, with a "b." Are these excesses healthy for our U.S. healthcare system?

Also consider the CEO of Aetna who retired in 2006 and who does not appear in Table 1.3. He has been chairman of the Board since April 1, 2001, and planned to also retire from that position at the end of 2006. In 2006, his salary was $1.1 million, his bonus was $2 million, and his other annual compensation was slightly more than $202,000. In addition, in 2006, he received 911,904 stock options and long-term compensation of over $4.5 million. Furthermore, according to the proxy statement, he owns or controls the equivalent of 6,338,393 shares of Aetna stock, just under 1 percent of the total shares outstanding. Is this former Aetna CEO another good example of insurance company excesses within the U.S. healthcare system? Would any health insurance policyholder or uninsured person approve of such overhead? Should any health insurance company board member allow such overhead to be heaped on policyholders?

Also consider the CEO of Caremark Rx, who earned $69.66 million in 2005, the ninth highest salary of any CEO in the United States. Caremark Rx, Inc., is a pharmaceutical services company that offers pharmacy benefit management services that involve the design and administration of programs for prescription drug use. The company dispenses pharmaceuticals to eligible participants.

Finally, consider the Humana CEO who also does not appear in Table 1.3. In 2005 he had total compensation of $2.6 million, which includes stock options. As of December 31, 2005, he held 1,088,621 exercisable stock options valued at $48 million and 449,996 unexercisable stock options valued at an additional $12.9 million. Is our U.S. health insurance system structured for profiteering or for delivering low cost quality care to patients?

A solution to eliminating insurance company excesses and overhead is to simply avoid these middlemen or at least rely less upon them. This may be done by expanding Medicare to cover more of the population and to somehow include coverage for children. Remember that Medicare adds a small 3 percent overhead to healthcare costs, compared to the 20 percent to 30 percent overhead added by insurance companies; a greater than 20 percent savings that would be more than

enough to pay for the 15.9 percent of Americans currently uninsured. Just eliminate the excess administrative costs of insurance
companies and one can then pay for the uninsured in America.
This is a logical and reasonable way to make U.S. healthcare more
affordable. It is one of the greatest and most obvious opportunities for shifting non-value-added dollars from insurance companies to providing true value-added healthcare services to patients
at lower cost.

Moving toward some kind of single-payer approach will also
greatly simplify complex dealings with thousands of different insurance companies, each with its own coverage rules. Even state-
sponsored programs like the ones recently enacted in Massachusetts
or Maine offer the promise of increasing coverage and reducing
costs. State programs, as in Illinois, that provide insurance to all
children are also gathering strong support. Other options extend the
insurance program available to government workers and legislators
to more of the U.S. population. Or, simply self-insuring a company
if it is large enough would direct more dollars to valued-added
patient care. Adopting a universal healthcare system for most of the
U.S. population would eliminate non-value-added insurance underwriting costs and mountains of unnecessary paperwork and administrative tasks. The goal is simply to direct a greater portion of
current health expenditures toward true value-added care for patients
as opposed to funding unnecessary overhead.

Remember our precept that the treatment of patients is primarily
between them and their physician and nurse(s) and supporting ancillary
departments, and yet large administrative support structures surround
them. Thirty-one cents of every dollar spent for healthcare in the
United States goes to administrative costs, according to an August 20,
2003 article in the *New England Journal of Medicine*.[18] That's nearly
double the rate in Canada. According to that article, the United States
spent $294 billion on healthcare paperwork and administration in 1999.
Having a U.S. delivery system administered as efficiently as the one in
Canada would save $209 billion annually, the authors say, enough to
insure all Americans who now lack health insurance.

In addition to Canada, other countries that have model single-
payer systems include France, Germany, and the Netherlands. These
single-payer systems standardize all the paperwork, greatly reduce
administrative costs, eliminate the underwriting and health insurance

application process, eliminate the patient payment process as they are funded by increased taxes, and provide a defined level of healthcare to each citizen. In our current insurance-based payment system, it is very common for a provider to have to file a claim for reimbursement multiple times before it is paid. In 2003, Maine became the first state to enact a single-payer health system for every resident. It is projected to save $1 billion by 2008, compared to Maine's 2004 health expenditures of $8.4 billion. The Maine system will also be able to negotiate statewide for better pharmaceutical prices. Maine plans to penalize pharmaceutical companies that refuse to sell drugs to uninsured people at the same discounted prices that Medicaid pays. Allowing the Medicare system to more aggressively negotiate drug costs with pharmaceutical companies was one of the goals of the Democrats following their landslide midterm election victory in November 2006. Such pharmaceutical savings will benefit many U.S. healthcare recipients. Shouldn't U.S. residents enjoy pharmaceutical savings comparable to those in Canada or other countries with universal healthcare, since we manufacture most of the drugs? By contrast, drug makers have begun a campaign to prevent Medicare negotiating low prices. Drug makers have not set a budget for their campaign, but they and their trade groups already spend $100 million a year on lobbying in Washington, a non-value added cost that could be better directed to actual patient care.

Streamlining payer methods will help reduce healthcare costs, but these do *nothing* to attack the other root cause, which is wasteful healthcare operating practices. Eliminating waste and overhead from healthcare processes is a huge opportunity to redirect savings to value-added patient care. It's clear there are plenty of opportunities to reduce healthcare costs. In this book, hospital executives can learn how Toyota lean production works and how to apply it to their organizations, and then they can then continuously lower cost and improve quality to reach board-approved goals.[19]

U.S. HEALTH EXPENDITURES ARE A GROWING PERCENTAGE OF GDP

According to the government-run Center for Medicare and Medicaid Services, total U.S. national personal healthcare expenditures were

$1.3 trillion in calendar year 2000, or nearly 14 percent of the gross domestic product (GDP).[20] (This grew about 50 percent to approximately $2 trillion by 2006.) Of the 2000 total, $412 billion or 32 percent was for hospital services, $286 billion or 22 percent was for physician services, $122 billion or 9 percent was for prescriptions, and $92 billion or 7 percent was for nursing home service. *Hospitals by far account for the greatest percent (32 percent) of total national healthcare expenditures,* that is, nearly 1.5 times total physician expenses. Hospitals are the top priority, but all healthcare providers including physician practices, pharmaceutical companies, and nursing homes are candidates for lean improvements. Between 2001 and 2011, health spending is projected to grow 2.5 percent per year faster than GDP, so it will constitute 17 percent of GDP by 2012 (see Figure 1.7). It is interesting to note that France and Italy were ranked No. 1 and 2 in health system effectiveness by the World Health Organization, and they each spend only 8 percent to 10 percent of their GDP on healthcare.[21] It is also interesting that Italy, which has the third largest health system in Europe, behind Germany and France, spends 41 percent of its health expenditures on physicians, 18 percent on hospital care, and 11 percent on drugs. While drug expenditures are similar to the 9 percent of GDP spent in the United States, Italy spends far less on hospital care: 18 percent of GDP compared to 32 percent in the United States. This is consistent with a lean goal of saving one half. Conversely, Italy spends almost twice

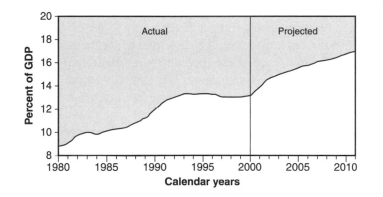

Figure 1.7 National health expenditures as a share of gross domestic product (GDP).

Source: CMS, Office of the Actuary, National Health Statistics Group.

as much on physicians, 41 percent of GDP compared to 22 percent in the United States. Back to our premise that a patient's care is primarily between them and their physician and nurse(s): Italy's greater proportion of funding for physicians makes sense because physicians, like nurses, are usually providing patients with value-added services.

A headline in *USA Today* reads, "Medicare system projected to go broke in 15 years," that is, by 2019, which is seven years earlier than previously predicted.[22]

A current report from the trustees of Medicare and Social Security blames this deterioration on "lower-than-expected revenue from workers' payroll taxes, higher spending on healthcare and the prescription drug benefit Congress passed in 2003." The report shows that the expenses for Medicare will exceed the revenue from payroll taxes and beneficiary premiums as soon as 2011. Clearly, some important changes are needed to reduce the cost of healthcare, reduce Medicare expenses, and/or increase Medicare funding.

U.S. SPENDS TWICE AS MUCH ON HEALTHCARE BUT RANKS 37TH IN HEALTH SYSTEM PERFORMANCE

The U.S. spends more than any other country per capita on healthcare. The U.S. spends per capita on healthcare nearly twice as much as each of the next highest spending countries of Switzerland, Norway, Germany, and Canada. Please see Figures 1.8, 1.9, and 1.10.[23] At the same time that U.S. health expenditures and insurance premiums continue rising at unprecedented rates, the quality of U.S. healthcare remains a serious issue. We're paying more but not necessarily getting better quality. According to a study by World Health Organization done in 2000, the U.S. ranked 37th in the world out of 191 countries in "health system performance," with France and Italy ranking first and second, even though they spend half as much per capita on healthcare. Based on key national performance indicators, U.S. healthcare is less cost effective than in 36 other countries. Please also note that U.S. pharmaceutical charges are increasing at the third fastest rate within OECD countries (Organization for Economic Cooperation & Development) even though most pharmaceutical

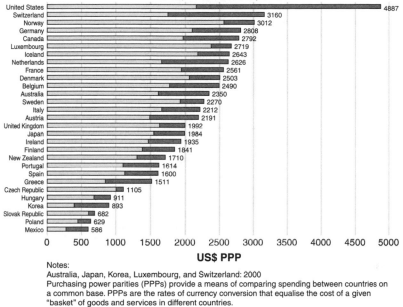

Notes:
Australia, Japan, Korea, Luxembourg, and Switzerland: 2000
Purchasing power parities (PPPs) provide a means of comparing spending between countries on a common base. PPPs are the rates of currency conversion that equalise the cost of a given "basket" of goods and services in different countries.

Figure 1.8   Health expenditure per capita, US$ PPP, 2001.

Source: OECD Health Data 2003.

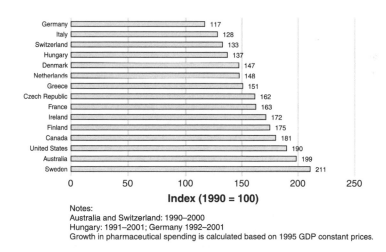

Notes:
Australia and Switzerland: 1990–2000
Hungary: 1991–2001; Germany 1992–2001
Growth in pharmaceutical spending is calculated based on 1995 GDP constant prices.

Figure 1.9   Growth in pharmaceutical expenditure per capita, in real terms, 1990–2001 (1990 = 100).

Source: OECD Health Data 2003.

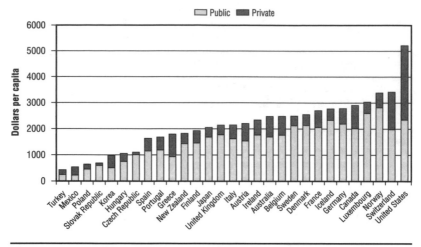

Figure 1.10 Public and private expenditure on health, U.S. dollars per capita, calculated using "purchasing power parities" (PPP), 2002.

companies are located in the United States (Figure 1.9). Surprisingly, the U.S. ranked 27th among industrialized countries for infant mortality rate, with 6.9 deaths per 1000 live births or .69 percent. This is nearly double the rate in Sweden, Finland, Norway, and Japan. One wonders if this might also be related to the epidemic of obesity in the United States.[24]

QUALITY PROBLEMS IN U.S. HEALTHCARE

30 Percent of Total U.S. Healthcare Costs Result from Poor Quality

The Midwest Business Group on Health estimates that 30 percent of total U.S. healthcare costs result from poor quality, defined as shown in Figure 1.11. This estimate is consistent with lean producers' claims to improve efficiency by 50 percent by removing waste and streamlining processes. The Chicago-based Midwest Business Group on Health (MBGH) was founded in January 1980 by a group of Midwestern employers to address escalating healthcare costs, which threatened

MBGH definition of poor quality includes:

- *Overuse.* A variety of surgical procedures, tests, medications, and treatments are overused, driving up costs unnecessarily while simultaneously exposing patients to risks of complication and sometimes even death.

- *Underuse.* Providers routinely fail to administer a variety of known-to-be-effective tests and treatments to heart attack victims and individuals with diabetes and congestive heart failure.

- *Misuse.* Medical errors represent the most common form of misuse within the healthcare system, with drug misuse representing the most frequent form of error.

- *Waste.* Waste, primarily in the form of unnecessary administrative activities, is prevalent throughout healthcare, as it is in many other industries.

Figure 1.11 The Midwest Business Group on Health estimates 30 percent of total costs results from poor-quality healthcare.

Source: Midwest Business Group on Health 2002

the competitiveness of U.S. employers and the welfare of their employees, families, and the population at large.[25]

Patients Typically Receive 55 Percent of Recommended Care

According to a study published in the *New England Journal of Medicine,* participating patients received 54.9 percent of the recommended care.[26] Based on this study, it is little different than a coin toss as to whether a patient will receive the recommended care for a given condition. The study involved telephoning a random sample of 13,275 adults in 12 metropolitan areas and asking them about their selected healthcare experiences. Investigators also received written consent to copy medical records for the most recent two-year period to evaluate performance based on 439 indicators of quality of care for 30 acute and chronic conditions as well as preventive care. Quality varied markedly by medical condition, ranging from a high of 78.7 percent of recommended care, delivered for senile cataract, to a low of 10.5 percent, delivered for alcohol dependence. This study concludes: "The deficits we have identified in adherence to recommended processes for basic care pose serious threats to the health of the American public. Strategies to reduce these deficits in care are warranted." This study provides strong support for better standardizing care processes, just as Toyota standardized its manufacturing process steps. (See step 27 on page 109.)

Building a Safer Health System

In its report, *To Err Is Human: Building a Safer Health System,* the Institute of Medicine states:

> Healthcare in the United States is not as safe as it should be and can be. At least 44,000 people, and perhaps as many as 98,000 people, die in hospitals each year as a result of medical errors that could have been prevented, according to estimates from two major studies. The knowledgeable health reporter for the *Boston Globe,* Betsy Lehman, died from an overdose during chemotherapy. Willie King had the wrong leg amputated. Ben Kolb was eight years old when he died during "minor" surgery due to a drug mix-up.[27]

These horrific cases that make the headlines are just the tip of the iceberg. Two large studies, one conducted in Colorado and Utah and the other in New York, found that adverse events occurred in 2.9 and 3.7 percent of hospitalizations, respectively. That is, approximately 1 in 21 patients experiences an adverse event during hospitalization.

The study in Colorado and Utah implies that at least 44,000 Americans die each year as a result of medical errors. The New York study suggests the number of deaths may be as high as 98,000.

Even when using the lower estimate, deaths due to medical errors represent the seventh leading cause of death in the United States. More people die in a given year as a result of medical errors than from motor vehicle accidents (43,458), breast cancer (42,297), or AIDS (16,516). Only a few hundred people die each year from airplane crashes. Think about that. The seventh leading cause of death in the U.S. is medical errors. Much more effort needs to be focused on reducing this horrendous statistic.

> *Medical errors* can be defined as the failure of a planned action to be completed as intended or the use of a wrong

plan to achieve an aim. Among the problems that commonly occur during the course of providing healthcare are adverse drug events and improper transfusions, surgical injuries and wrong-site surgery, suicides, restraint-related injuries or death, falls, burns, pressure ulcers, and mistaken patient identities. High error rates with serious consequences are most likely to occur in intensive care units, operating rooms, and emergency departments. Beyond their cost in human lives, preventable medical errors exact other significant tolls. They have been estimated to result in total costs (including the expense of additional care necessitated by the errors, lost income and household productivity, and disability) of between $17 billion and $29 billion per year in hospitals nationwide.[28]

It is not sufficient to address excessive medical errors by just adding more staff and more costs. Rather it is important to get at the root causes of errors, and to design systems that make the errors impossible to occur. (See poka-yoke techniques on page 90.)

Healthcare providers need to adopt an important technique from the aerospace industry called failure mode and effects analysis (FMEA) to reduce errors in healthcare. FMEA originated in the 1960s to improve safety in the aerospace and chemical industries. The goal of FMEA is to prevent safety accidents from ever occurring. This is precisely what we wish to accomplish within healthcare. Automotive and other industries have similarly adopted FMEA analyses, and it's time for the healthcare industry to do likewise. This simple FMEA technique can help reduce the 98,000 medically related deaths and billions in unnecessary costs annually.[29]

The steps within a FMEA analysis can be a simple process as follows:

1. Perform a detailed review of the product or process. A team may be used.

2. Brainstorm all ways the process can fail, that is, all failure modes.

3. List the potential effects of each failure mode.

4. Assign a 1–10 Severity rating for each effect.
   10 = highest

5. Assign a 1–10 probability of Occurrence rating for each failure mode. 10 = highest probability.

6. Assign a 1–10 Detection rating for each failure mode and/or effect. 10 = not detectable.

7. Calculate the risk priority number (RPN) for each effect. For example, Severity # × Occurrence # × Detection #. Add them all together to get the total RPN for all effects related to a given failure mode.

8. Prioritize the failure modes for action via the RPN score. (That is, list the failure modes in decreasing order by RPN score.)

9. Take action to eliminate or reduce the high RPN failure modes.

10. Calculate the resulting RPN as the failure modes are reduced or eliminated. These new RPN scores should be zero or at least now highly reduced.

PAST FAILURE OF CONTINUOUS QUALITY IMPROVEMENT AND TOTAL QUALITY MANAGEMENT

In the past, both continuous quality improvement (CQI) and total quality management (TQM) have been used for improvement in healthcare and elsewhere.

CQI is a process of continuously making everything better each day. It is customer focused and requires that processes be analyzed, measured, and improved on an ongoing basis. It has essentially failed in healthcare in the past because it was not implemented widely or continuously throughout organizations. Rather, it occurs sporadically every four years just before inspections by the Joint Commission for Accreditation of Healthcare Organizations (JCAHO). CQI has basically failed to markedly improve overall cost and quality in healthcare. It has not involved most healthcare employees, and rarely has it been focused on cost.

TQM is a management system in which everyone within an organization constantly monitors what they do to find ways of improving quality of operations, products, services, marketing, customer and employee satisfaction, and everything else. It is a broader concept that includes CQI. Every individual is responsible for improving the quality of goods and services supplied. Ford with its "Quality is Job One" slogan illustrates this organizationwide philosophy. Again, TQM has basically failed in healthcare organizations in the past since employees simply didn't understand it. Like CQI, it has not been pervasive throughout organizations, and it has been intermittently applied. It too has been rarely focused on cost in healthcare.

Basically CQI and TQM approaches were done to satisfy JCAHO requirements and have not moved healthcare organizations toward world-class levels of low cost and high quality. CQI and TQM have not generally been the primary focus of hospital boards. A new approach in which hospital boards, administrators, and all staff continuously focus on improving healthcare cost and quality is needed. For this to occur, they must receive adequate rewards and/or negative consequences, or the status quo will continue or degenerate.

REDESIGNING THE U.S. HEALTHCARE SYSTEM

If a reasonable person were to redesign a new U.S. healthcare system from scratch, they would not likely come up with anything like the present system (or should we say nonsystem). The system we have has evolved over the last 200 years, from its beginnings as a cottage industry. Early healthcare providers grew independently within a generally noncoordinated system of similar healthcare providers that have become more like a patchwork quilt than a designed system. If designed in a logical manner, each healthcare provider would serve a limited population in a defined geographic area without duplication. Smaller, satellite centers would refer patients to larger centers to address more difficult cases. The most difficult cases at large centers would be addressed by regional and national centers with extensive capabilities and specialty expertise. A logically designed national healthcare system would look more like a tree with satellite centers as its small branches, regional centers as its large branches, and national centers as its trunk. All costs and charges would be uniform across the United States except for small cost of living adjustments. Possibly there should be a law that all hospital charges be equal to the appropriate Medicare charge + X percent. In fact, the Medical Savings Insurance Company of Oklahoma and Indiana in 2004 sued certain Florida hospitals that were refusing to accept its routine payments of Medicare charges plus 20 percent for treatment of any non-Medicare patients.[30]

In a well-designed system, all patients would also have uniform access to services, and duplication would be minimized within each service area. To move in that direction, some states require a hospital to complete a "certificate of need" before new construction is approved. However, that is not required in many states. At a minimum, our government should institute a national certificate of need process for all healthcare providers, to make services uniformly available across the nation and evenly distribute costs. Our current system, which has run amok, is more like a garden overgrown with varieties of plants and weeds. Each plant and weed tries to overtake the other in an uncontrolled erratic manner. What determines which one survives is more a matter of warring factions, that is, the strongest survives, than any logical design to achieve specific community goals of cost and quality.[31]

The United States will sooner or later need to coordinate its nonsystem of healthcare. A national imperative is for our country to create a target design for an ideal healthcare delivery system and to create incentives for all stakeholders to begin to gradually move from the nonsystem toward that ideal design. Maybe it's time to create a new Spartan but highly functional hospital design that provides good nurse staffing; good access to competent physician(s) who attend patients; and good ancillary lab, x-ray, and pharmacy services. All of this would be contained in a compact, low-cost facility that eliminates all other services that a patient does not wish to personally pay for. Maybe it's time to construct a hospital model that is simply centered on the patient, his or her physicians, nurses, and critical ancillary functions and that contains little or no excess overhead. This ideally designed healthcare system would also minimize handoffs of the patient among too many physicians and hospital staff. How can a patient receive high-quality care if it involves too many participants who aren't comparing notes? A similar streamlined design may be considered for any other type of healthcare provider, for example, clinic, nursing home, or rehab center.

2

Respect for Employees

The immediate key to stopping the rise in healthcare costs is to eliminate all forms of waste in healthcare. This can be started now without any new legislation. However, wholesale "re-engineering" or "downsizing" efforts create extreme ill will and must be avoided at all costs. It is critical for hospital administrators to create an environment of trust and honesty, employee community, and mutual respect. Dr. W. Edwards Deming aptly stated this idea as one of his quality improvement principles: "Drive out fear, build trust." Deming also stated that 80% of problems are related to management or systems. Similarly Taiichi Ohno, father of the Toyota Production System, focused on "respect for humanity" as one of his guiding principles for building a lean, low-cost, high-quality production system. Peter Drucker contended that each organization has a major goal of personal growth for its employees. After World War II, Japan tried to maintain long-term employment (lifetime employment) for core personnel, whose experiences were important assets to Japanese companies. We should show the same high ethical standards toward all employees while rebuilding the U.S. healthcare system. It's important to base management decisions on a long-term view of developing and retaining dedicated and valuable employees even at the expense of short-term financial goals. Promote the concept of the "family of employees," with its members truly receiving earned respect. These employees will then faithfully commit long term to providing value-added services to patients and customers. From within, grow leaders and high-performing employees who are committed to the organization. Michael Hammer, the renowned reengineering expert, stated in one of his reengineering training videos that the soft stuff is the hard stuff. He explained that any problem that could be mathematically described was essentially an easy problem compared to motivational and value alignment issues with employees, where the greatest opportunities and benefits reside. Take a long-term view of aligning all employees toward common goals. Protect the knowledge in the organization through these committed employees.

Employers, particularly in healthcare, have a responsibility to their existing employees as they pursue "lean production" or any other quality improvement/cost reduction strategy, such as reengineering, Six Sigma, or TQM. At the beginning of a lean implementation, it's a good idea to announce that no layoffs will result from these efforts. Otherwise, the employees will be reluctant to cooperate fully. The Toyota plant in Fremont, California, has both no-layoff and no-strike clauses in its union contract to foster continuous improvement and cost reduction. Each healthcare administrator has an ethical responsibility to do everything in his or her power to retain all employees who are functioning at a defined level of good performance. If necessary, a hiring freeze should be implemented early on to retain and, if necessary, redeploy good employees instead of hiring new employees. Attrition or voluntary early retirement may also be used to move toward leaner processes. If job changes occur as a result of cost reduction and process improvement, let existing employees know up front that they will be preferred over new hires for any new positions that become available and for which they are qualified.

Respect each employee as an important contributor to improvement of quality, cost, and the organization itself. Creating an environment of respect for the employee is the core around which a successful lean production system is built. Everyone's ideas, suggestions, and opinions are equally important.

Part II

Reduce Healthcare Cost and Improve Quality by Using Toyota Lean Production Methods

3

46 Steps to Improve Cost and Quality in the U.S. Healthcare System

I will continue by dealing primarily with reducing the cost and improving the quality of healthcare processes. If we improve each of the detailed process steps in how we deliver healthcare, we can thus improve overall healthcare cost and quality. The following methods are primarily the same methods used by Toyota Motor Company and other "lean producers." This book won't further pursue the "macro" system for financing the delivery of healthcare. It also won't further talk about HMOs, PPOs, Medicare, Medicaid, or other payer systems. Those subjects are highly politically charged on their own. Instead, I will address "process improvement methods" that may be applied to any healthcare system regardless of payer.[1] I acknowledge that the aging of America and the introduction of new and better technologies are contributing to higher health insurance premiums, but there is little doubt that healthcare processes themselves can be made much more efficient and cost effective.

It took Toyota 30 years to achieve world-class success through its lean production methods. Similarly, lean is not an overnight solution to U.S. healthcare cost and quality problems. Rather, lean is a multi-year strategic direction for healthcare providers to adopt. Improvement then continues in a never-ending fashion toward the elusive goal of "perfection." A valuable exercise for healthcare providers is to develop a strategic plan for lean by mapping each of the 46 steps that follow into for example a three- to five-year implementation plan.

I now present the following 46 steps to improve healthcare cost and quality based on Toyota Lean Production methods, the advice of lean advocates and quality experts such as W. Edwards Deming, Peter Drucker, Joseph Juran, Philip Crosby, Taiichi Ohno, Shigeo Shingo, Iwao Kobayashi, James Womack, Don Berwick, and also my own 30 years of experience with process improvement in healthcare.

 # Define Value from the Perspective of the Patient (Customer)

Value from the patient's perspective means easy access to appointments, no wait times, timely reports, timely decisions, good outcomes, courtesy, reasonable costs, and so forth. A technical definition for a "value-added task" is one that satisfies all of the following:

- It is an activity

- It is requested by or important to the patient (that is, something the patient is willing to personally pay for)

- It changes the thing being processed

- It is done right the first time (that is, without any rework or waste)

Use focus groups and surveys to clarify exactly what patients define as value to themselves. When was the last time you asked a patient about the quality and cost of their care? Find out what, when, where, and how much the patient actually requires versus what is actually being delivered. Would an uninsured patient choose to pay for a particular process step, activity, or feature? If not, consider eliminating it. Does building a fancy new healthcare facility that looks like the Taj Mahal provide true value to the patient? Does that expensive fountain in the lobby provide true value to the patient, especially one of the 46 million uninsured? Do expanded hospital services provide true value to the patient and community even if similar, high-quality services are already available at a nearby hospital? What is the primary goal of a healthcare provider? Is it to increase its bottom line and market share?

Or should the true goal be to cost-effectively and measurably improve the health status of the community? How do we properly align the goals of neighboring hospital systems? Hospital boards and top executives need to do some soul searching to answer these questions.

It would be wise for key healthcare leaders to meet periodically with their competitors, and ask the question "How can we cooperatively serve the patients in our region more cost effectively?" It might begin with a transport bus that is jointly funded to visit most major providers in a region. There could be a shared ambulance and helicopter agreement designed to take the patient to the nearest appropriate healthcare site, as has been done in Seattle, Washington. Or, there might be a common, machine-readable patient ID card with insurance and demographic information to speed a patient's visit to any provider. It might progress toward noncompeting centers of excellence at each competitor with the competitors literally referring to one another. One competitor might say, "We'll focus on these centers of excellences, and compete less with you as you focus on those." Or, "This piece of new equipment is extremely expensive. Is there a way to possibly use just one for the benefit of all patients in the region?" Based on commitment and cooperation, it is possible for a shared affordable healthcare vision to become a reality.

 ## Map the Patient's Value Stream

A patient's *value stream* is defined as "all of the actions, both value-creating and non-value-creating, required to bring the patient from admission through discharge and follow-up. A value-stream map is a diagram identifying all the activities needed to receive, care for, discharge, and follow a patient. These include actions to process information for the patient and actions to transform the patient toward a desired outcome. A value stream may be mapped as a flow-chart of process steps and as a block diagram showing the relation of all physical locations and objects involved. The actions within a patient value-stream map can be divided into three categories: those that definitely provide patient value, those that provide business value but little or no patient value, and those that provide no value whatsoever. Once the patient's value stream is mapped, the challenge is to provide the patient with value-added steps while removing all non-value-added steps and minimizing all business value-added steps. Ask whether a patient without health insurance would likely choose to pay for a particular step. If not, try to eliminate it. Improvement goals include eliminating waiting times, streamlining meetings, minimizing inventories, and minimizing transport wherever possible, such as for all patients, staff, procedures, and all supplies. Consider putting a pedometer on a typical patient or staff member, record the transport distance, and then minimize it. Transport is inherently non-value-added and must be reduced or eliminated wherever possible. (See step 25 for more on eliminating waste.)

One tool that Toyota uses to improve a value stream is called an A3 form. Interestingly, the A3 improvement form is named after the large paper size (approximately 11 × 17 inches) that is typically used to draw it. Basically, the current condition or value stream is drawn on the left side of sheet. All of the issues, background, problems, and opportunities are listed. Then an improved future condition or new value-stream map is drawn on the right side, which contains all the target improvements. Also, list the implementation plan, that is, the steps needed to reach the target condition. This includes the countermeasures that need to be taken to overcome issues to reach the target condition. The A3 form is a simple and concise high-level problem-solving approach that fits on a single sheet of paper. Figure 3.1 is a sample A3 report format.

3 Walk Through All Your Core Processes, and Observe How They Work in Detail

Go see your employees' work process for yourself. Understand their work processes thoroughly, even if it means observing for days. Numbers will never substitute for the understanding of actually being there. Consider actually performing the jobs yourself if possible to

ISSUE	TARGET CONDITION	TITLE
BACKGROUND		TO
		BY
CURRENT CONDITION		DATE
	COUNTERMEASURES	
	IMPLEMENTATION PLAN	
	what who when outcome	
PROBLEM ANALYSIS		
	COST COST BENEFIT/WASTE RECOGNITION	
	TEST	
	FOLLOW UP	

Figure 3.1 A3 form.

further increase your understanding. Require that supervisors and managers periodically do the actual value-added work, so that they are intimately familiar with all operations and can identify the steps that don't add value. Personally verify relevant data. Then let everyone think, speak about, and improve processes from personally verified experience and observations. Even high-level managers, vice presidents, and presidents should periodically observe processes in detail, target improvements, and then verify that the improvements are achieved and maintained. Seriously consider creating an internal observation team that includes the manager or supervisor of an area along with selected employees and improvement facilitators. Create this observation and improvement team from internal staff, as opposed to using expensive external consultants. Focus on removing the waste (muda) and creating continuous flow. You will be amazed by what you see if you just take the time to look carefully.

4 Implement Toyota-Style Lean Production Methods

Establish a continuous flow of work and eliminate delays and waits wherever possible. Clearly state a goal of cutting patient waiting time to zero or at least target a maximum wait-time standard. Post that standard in all areas: for example, "If you have been waiting more than 20 minutes, please inform the front desk person." With patients flowing more steadily and smoothly through treatment areas, the size of waiting rooms and even the treatment areas themselves may be reduced. Continuous flow minimizes patient wait time and treatment time. Likewise, strive to reduce to zero the amount of time any patient or patient-related work project is sitting idle. Wherever possible, implement continuous flow for all patients, supplies, materials, process steps, and work projects. Continuous flow will quickly bring process problems to the surface for quick resolution.

It may be important to use a high-quality, coordinated scheduling system to control smooth patient flow throughout the entire organization. Effective patient scheduling is one way in which computer technology is well applied. Investing in efficient patient scheduling is likely to be an investment in efficiency. However, analyze the situation carefully because a simple "pull system" that essentially moves the patient through treatment steps may even simplify scheduling. A pull system is one in which patients (customers) pulls value (toward themselves) from preceding upstream activities. So, if the patients need a major activity performed on them, that need would automatically pull all required resources and value directly to the patients. The patients should quickly draw all needed services as they move through their treatment experience. A pull system will provide patients with what they want, when they want it, and in the amount they want. Recognize that Toyota does not use a sophisticated scheduling system when moving automobiles through the manufacturing process. Instead the automobiles move smoothly between each process step with all supplies and inventory provided just in time via the use of kanbans, which are discussed in step 25.7. So, wherever you can create a simple pull system to efficiently move patients through their treatments, that is preferred over complex or automated scheduling systems.

A novel kanban card may be used for patients being treated and can immediately pull services to that patient at each step in the treatment. For example, a receptionist can give an identifying (kanban) card (with the patient's ID number written on it) to the patient upon arrival at the reception desk. After an x-ray is complete, the patient returns the card to the receptionist. The card is then a signal for the receptionist to immediately notify the doctor to see the patient (since the x-ray is already viewable over the digital x-ray system). This signal for the physician to see the patient is automatic without the need to repeatedly ask additional questions of the patient or staff, such as patient name and so forth. This use of a simple card (kanban) can quickly and easily draw many other services immediately to a patient as he or she moves through each of the tests and treatments. Again, this can be done without a costly computerized tracking system.

Please also recognize that patient care paths are designed to pull value to the patient in a scheduled manner. Scrutinize each care path so that its execution becomes nearly automatic, that is, it automatically and continuously pulls value to the patient. The additional steps that follow expand on the methods used to create a lean production system.

5 Train Administrators, Managers, and Supervisors to be Lean Leaders

What does it mean for a supervisor, manager, or administrator to be a lean leader? Lean leaders focus on quality, service, price, and both customer and employee satisfaction. They keep removing non-value-added steps, waste, and waiting time and allow value to be continuously pulled to the customer. They relentlessly improve to assure future growth, market share, and profit. They manage with great respect and empathy as if they personally owned part of the business.

Being a lean leader means he or she respects the potential contribution and knowledge of every employee, especially frontline workers. Frontline employees best know the problems they face every day, and they usually know best how to solve them. It means giving employees the latitude to improve their own work to establish better standardized processes. It means engaging every employee touching a value stream to sustain and improve flow. It means promoting experimentation, tolerating failures, and learning from them to eventually produce world-class results. It means assigning a leader to each value stream with the responsibility to continuously improve it. This leader will make the current condition of the value stream clear to everyone, propose an improved future state, take responsibility to make it happen, make the condition of the newly improved value stream clear to everyone, and then repeat this sequence over and over, striving for perfection. Most managers think vertically to optimize their own department or function, while a value-stream manager thinks horizontally to optimize the ultimate value to the patient/customer. Negotiation occurs between value-stream managers and vertical managers to optimize customer value together. Together they also develop beneficial career paths for employees.

But how do these managers and administrators lead the transition to lean? They do this by getting each employee to think and take initiative to improve his or her own job, and they ensure that these continual improvements add value for customers. Together with employees they strive for a system that delivers the best quality, lowest cost, and shortest lead times. They provide what is needed just in time (JIT) where it is needed, maintain continuous workflow at a steady acceptable rate, and use pull systems to quickly provide services to the patient or customer. They build quality into each step of the process by quickly correcting any defective process—they ask "why" five times to get at the true root cause of defects. Together, they mistake-proof processes and use visual controls, well-organized work places, and total maintenance to keep equipment always productive. They maintain a steady workflow that is easily manageable for all and avoid overloading anyone. They guard against excessive variation. They minimize defects. They treat suppliers as partners with a common goal of increasing value to the patient or customer. They rely upon teams of cross-trained employees with team leaders and group leaders above them. A lean leader's job is to develop his or her own people, and they lead "as though they themselves have no power." They rely heavily on employees' taking responsibility or they say, "Let's figure this out together." They focus on continual process improvement both in cost and quality, and they avoid finger pointing and blame. They expect problems to occur, and they know that masking, hiding, or burying problems from sight is the biggest kind of problem. Their goal is to expose problems so that they are quickly and permanently corrected. A lean system is inherently designed to identify and positively respond to problems. A lean system is a flexible system rather than a controlling system.

Lean administrators are visibly committed to lean improvement. They regularly spend time on the floor to see how well things are actually working. They do this often. When was the last time you asked the staff about and observed how well processes were actually working? Lean administrators, managers, supervisors, and employees continually support kaizen improvement efforts that may each last from a day to a month. They demonstrate "empathetic change management" and do their best to accommodate any employee who appears adversely affected by a transition to lean. The lean foundation of respect for employees, committed executive leadership, continual improvement, and empathetic change management keeps the lean journey as vibrant as it has been with Toyota. Senior leaders provide the vision and incentive, middle managers help design and implement the lean changes, and frontline workers make them happen daily.[2]

QUALITIES OF LEAN LEADERS

- Build 46 steps into their 3 to 5 year strategic plan to improve quality and cost.

- Focus on continual process improvement.

- Regularly spend time in the department seeing.

- Assign a leader to each core process to improve it. Expose problems and improve flow.

- Respect and encourage employee contribution.

- Rely heavily on employees to take responsibility. Develop employees.

- Focus on processes and avoid blame.

- Provide empathetic change management.

HOW DO EMPLOYEES MAKE IMPROVEMENT HAPPEN?

- Continually improve own work (flow) to add value for patient/customer.

- Participate in Rapid Improvement Events.

- Help the patient/customer pull value.

- Standardize processes.

- Stop and correct defective processes to reduce future defects. Expose problems.

- Help mistake proof processes.

- Make lots of suggestions for improvement.

Provide Empathetic "Change Management" to Ease the Transition to Lean

Employees will alter their mind-sets only if they see the point of the change and agree with it—at least enough to give it a try. The surrounding structures (reward and recognition systems, for example) must be in tune with the new behavior. Employees must have the skills to do what is required. Finally, they must see people they respect acting as role models. Each of these conditions: 1) seeing the need for change, 2) surrounding structures, 3) requisite employee skills, and 4) leadership, is realized independently. Together they add up to a way of changing the behavior of people in organizations by changing attitudes about what can and should happen at work.

Unsurprisingly, the above conditions map very nicely to model that we in the Theory of Constraints community refer to as the Six Layers of Resistance to buy-in. . . .

Layer One—Lack of agreement on the problem.

Layer Two—Lack of agreement on a direction for a solution.

Layer Three—Lack of agreement that the solution addresses the full problem.

Layer Four—Concerns regarding side effects of the solution.

Layer Five—Concerns regarding obstacles to implementation of the solution.

Layer Six—Unspoken fears.

Defining and implementing a solution requires knowing not just the technical aspects of the problem, but also bringing stakeholders and necessary participants through the Six Layers. In the McKinsey article[3], the first condition of seeing the point of the change and agreeing with it sufficiently starts to get through the first four resistance layers. Without agreement on a problem, there's no point talking about a change. Even if everyone recognizes the problem, it may be so ingrained that it's seen as the nature of doing what we do, with no real way of dealing with it. A direction is one thing, but if people are going to agree with it, a whole lot of communication is needed. Finally, if one sees the proposed solution as a possible prelude to something worse, there will be foot dragging.

The second condition of the article[3]—having surrounding structures "in tune" with the new policies, processes, and desired behaviors—reflects some of the needed communication. New policies, metrics, and rewards are necessary to ensure that the desired behaviors are achieved. Condition three—employee skills or, rather, the lack of necessary skills—is one of the obstacles of layer five.

Finally, one of the toughest layers of resistance, if it appears, is number six—unspoken fear, often fear of going it alone. Especially for changes that involve considerable culture change—major changes in behavior—being the first out of the trenches and out into no-man's-land can be a daunting experience. While the first five resistance layers can be largely dealt with through clarity of thought and communication, the best means of moving people out of their fear is through leadership. Leadership is, as the McKinsey article suggests, role modeling and supporting desired behaviors. (Note that much of the text in step 6 above was excerpted from the McKinsey article[3].)

Change "Quality Improvement Department" to "Quality and Cost Improvement Department"

This new Quality and Cost Improvement Department will help stop skyrocketing healthcare costs. Merge the past Quality Improvement Department with any existing industrial or management engineering functions, decision support/data analysis functions, and performance improvement education functions into a single, newly named Quality and Cost Improvement department. To help stop skyrocketing

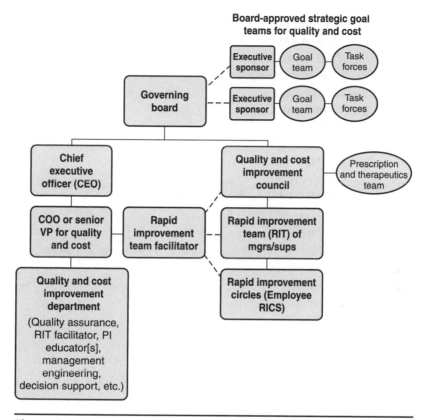

Figure 3.2 Organizational structure for quality and cost improvement.

healthcare costs, this newly named department will focus equally on improving both cost and quality. Change the name of the hospital's main Quality Council that reports to the board of directors to Quality and Cost Improvement Council. This Quality and Cost Improvement Council will create a vision of continuous improvement for the entire organization and meet at least monthly to solidly and visibly support that vision, create a policy and procedure statement for the improvement process, publish a new Quality and Cost Improvement Manual, and suggest objectives for future employee teams. The Quality and Cost Improvement Council, in concert with the hospital board, will set objective cost and quality goals at least yearly. Those will include goals such as "There will be no hospital cost increase this year" or, even more commendably, "We will achieve our quality objectives, and simultaneously reduce cost per CMI adjusted patient discharge by 5 percent per year for the next five years." Restructure cost and quality related departments and committees as shown in Figure 3.2. The roles of the Rapid Improvement Team (RIT) and Rapid Improvement Circles (RICs) of employees are more fully explained in steps 15 and 17.

8 Change the Name "Quality Improvement Manual" to "Quality and Cost Improvement Manual"

This manual will not only present quality improvement techniques but also cost improvement techniques for use throughout the organization.

9 Educate Every Employee About the Basic Strategic Plan of the Organization

It's easy to give each employee a business card that summarizes the organization's current strategic objectives. One side of the card should be used to record the employee's individual objectives (which are in fact aligned with the organization's objectives). An annual brochure may clarify the organization's mission, values, and organizational and individual strategic objectives. Each objective should have a what, when, why, how, and by whom description. In addition, I recommend displaying the organization's mission, values, and strategic objectives for each employee to see in the cafeteria and as they log in to any computer. By having every employee understand the organization's mission, values, and strategic objectives, and how their own objectives align with them, everyone is moving in the same direction. Visibly and orally share these items frequently among all employees.

10

Establish an Improvement Plan with Goals to be Accomplished by Specific People and Dates

Incorporate parts of this improvement plan into your organization's strategic plan. The hospital's main Quality and Cost Improvement Council should approve this improvement plan and its objectives and due dates. The hospital board should also receive a copy of this plan for its review and approval. Patient focus groups and survey results would strongly influence the direction of this plan. A Toyota plant has a clear goal that is shared by all, such as to be Number 1 in class in class in the next J. D. Powers survey. Similarly, a hospital may have related Baldrige, ISO 9000, JCAHO, or benchmarking achievement goals. A healthcare provider's plan may focus on improving specific areas and core processes such as:
(PVA = patient value added; BVA = business value added)

10.1	Staff scheduling to match patient loads (PVA)
10.2	Productivity monitoring (BVA)
10.3	Core process improvement
10.3.1	Admission (BVA)
10.3.2	Emergency room treatment (PVA)
10.3.3	All patient scheduling processes (BVA), such as inpatient and outpatient
10.3.4	Outpatient treatment (PVA)
10.3.5	Ancillary testing, such as lab and x-ray (PVA)
10.3.6	Surgical treatment (PVA)
10.3.7	Medical treatment (PVA)
10.3.8	Nursing care process (PVA)
10.3.9	Therapy treatments (PVA)
10.3.10	Medication process (PVA)
10.3.11	Discharge (BVA)

10.3.12   Billing (BVA)

10.4   Pharmaceutical cost reduction (PVA)

10.5   Defect reduction, such as med errors, infections, falls, medical procedure errors, and billing errors (PVA)

10.6   Supplies and materials cost reduction, such as inventory reduction and improved control (PVA)

10.7   Idealized design of physician office practices (PVA)

10.8   Rapid improvement team goals and initiatives (PVA)

10.9   Patient access to services throughout the region (PVA)

10.10   Strategic initiatives to support quality and cost improvement (PVA)

10.11   Organizational redesign of supervisory and administrative structures (BVA)

10.12   Minimizing financial losses in typically non-profitable departments (BVA)

10.13   Cost effective facility design and management (PVA/BVA)

10.14   Information systems redesign to support quality and cost improvement goals (PVA/BVA)

When improving a healthcare system, it is important to look at the entire patient experience. For example, map the value stream all the way from the recognition of a patient problem in a physician's office through scheduling their hospital admission, actual admission, treatment, discharge, billing, and payment, and even follow-up care. By improving the entire process of initial patient access through payment and follow-up, one increases the likelihood of a positive patient experience and bottom line results. Consider that a patient may have significant delay from the recognition of a medical need thru diagnosis and hospital admission. Also, a hospital stay may average 4 days, but receiving payment may take an additional 60 days. By looking at the whole process from recognition of medical need in the physician's office through discharge and payment received, one is able to improve the entire patient experience and positively affect the bottom line. This may also be done in a Pareto fashion by identifying the "highest value" diagnoses and procedures that can produce the greatest benefit if those value streams are improved. For example, it may be of greatest benefit to first look at the value streams of cardiac or orthopedic patients if one is attempting to achieve best "bottom line" financial improvements. Possibly improving the outpatient, emergency patient, or surgical patient value streams will also provide high benefit. When trying to improve a healthcare delivery system it is important to not just do "random acts of lean" all over and hope for optimal "bottom line" financial improvement. Focusing on high value "core services and processes" from point of access through payment received will produce targeted high value results.

11 Implement a Simple Scorecard for the Entire Healthcare Organization

Use a simple scorecard to monitor cost and quality improvement in the entire organization, and to "hold the gains." This scorecard is designed to show how efficiently the healthcare provider is operating in terms of numbers of patients seen, staffing provided, and cost per patient.

There are many queuing situations in which patients arrive and are serviced by staff. Be sure to maintain variable staffing in these areas so that when peak patient loads dissipate, you reduce staff accordingly. I have seen reception areas with possibly five receptionists and few or no patients after 2 P.M. or 3 P.M., or very light loads on certain days of the week like Friday. It's important to know the average patient load per day of the week, hour of the day, and month of the year so that you can staff appropriately. Too many healthcare providers overlook variable staffing opportunities, which can save large labor costs.[4]

A simple daily scorecard is shown in Figure 3.3. Strive to keep all your key performance reports to just one or two pages long, even for financial indicators. Quality indicators such as medical

Hospital Daily Staffing Report—Week Starting _____							
	Sun	Mon	Tue	Wed	Thur	Fri	Sat
1. Census							
Med/Surg							
Obstetrics							
ICU							
Nursery							
Total							
2. Visits							
Emergency							
Surgery							
L&D							
Total							
3. Total Nonproductive FTEs							
Med/Surg							
Obstetrics							
ICU							
Nursery							
Emergency							
Surgery							
L&D							
Nursing Admin.							
Total							
4. Total Productive FTEs							
Med/Surg							
Obstetrics							
ICU							
Nursery							
Emergency							
Surgery							
L&D							
Nursing Admin.							
Total							
5. Staffing Variences							
Over/Under FTE							
Med/Surg							
Obstetrics							
ICU							
Nursery							
Emergency							
Surgery							
L&D							
Nursing Admin.							
Total							
6. Ave. Cost/Day of Over/Under Staffing							
Dollars							
7. FTEs/Occupied Bed							

Figure 3.3 Hospital daily staffing report.

errors/incidents/defects may be added as second page to the score-card. This daily scorecard may be a simple spreadsheet that is available online for all to see. It can quickly show where the organization needs to take daily corrective action to improve cost and quality. Graphical monitoring may be added.[5] Also, consider sending each individual patient report of a hospital acquired infection or med error/incident/defect to the CEO, and then work as a team to minimize them. Each such error warrants immediate action to prevent any recurrence.

12 Use a Simple Scorecard to Monitor Each Department

Use a simple scorecard to periodically (for example, monthly) monitor the level of cost and quality within each department, service, or process to be improved. Figure 3.4 illustrates a scorecard that has the major headings of volume, productivity, quality, and cost. Also, roll multiple departmental scorecards monthly into a single hospitalwide scorecard. Consider adding the six performance indicators recommended by Goldratt, which are further discussed in improvement step 28. Also include the percentage of salaries for direct value-added caregivers divided by total salaries to reflect the portion of salaries going to direct value-added patient care. Flag results requiring immediate action in red, marginal results in yellow, and acceptable results in green.

Each department/service can easily maintain this type of scorecard using a spreadsheet program, such as Excel, or by using a paper form as shown in Figure 3.4. Each scorecard should fit on one or two pages to keep it simple. You may adapt the departmental scorecard to record measurements monthly, weekly, or daily depending on the nature of the improvements desired. The scorecard may be posted or displayed online where every employee can see it. This supports the Toyota principle of "visual control," in which all the processes and important parameters of a working department are visible to the workers.

Measurement and inspection are inherently not value added and are not necessary if the organization, department, service, product, or

Indicators	Target	Jul	Aug	Sep	Oct	Nov	Dec	etc.
1. Volume								
A. Avg. Daily Census								
B. Avg. Daily Procedure Count								
C. Avg. Daily Visits (Outpatient)								
2. Productivity								
A. Productive Hrs. Care per Day								
B. Productive Hrs Care per Procedure								
C. FTEs/Occupied Bed								
3. Quality								
A. No. of defects / Med Errors / Infections / Falls, etc.								
B. No. of incident reports								
C. Lawsuits								
D. $ Cost of A+B+C								
E. Patient Satisfaction Results								
4. Cost								
A. Cost per CMI Adjusted Discharge								
B. Avg. Cost per Patient Day								
C. Avg. Cost per Procedure								
D. Percent Understaffed or Overstaffed								
E. Cost of Understaffing or Overstaffing								
F. Total Patient Value Added Hours								
G. Total Hours worked								
H. Ratio of F/G %								
I. Total Patient Value-added Salary $								
J. Total Salary $								
K. Ratio of I/J %								

Figure 3.4 Departmental scorecard.

process works as designed every time. A patient would generally not want to pay for the effort it takes to monitor a process and might rightly expect the process to be done right the first time and every time. However, for those things that don't work perfectly every time, we need a scorecard to improve them and to then verify that we have improved them. It's key to focus on sustained improvement rather than just measurement. After we are comfortable that the newly improved department, service, product, or process is working consistently in the way we want, we can use the scorecard less frequently (quarterly or yearly) to ensure that operations haven't deteriorated. Or, we can eliminate certain scorecards or indicators completely if we have full confidence that the improvements are "built-in to last."

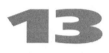 ## The Board of Directors Initiates Selected Strategic Quality and Cost Improvement Goals

In reality some managers and supervisors may heartily believe they already have a "lean staff" and may see process improvement projects as a "superfluous thing." Some may feel that process improvement is not a high priority compared to their day-to-day management and "firefighting" activities. A good way to overcome this reluctance is for the organization's board of directors to initiate selected "strategic quality and cost improvement goals" annually. For example, the board may identify and approve six or more strategic quality and cost goals for the year. The board appoints a senior executive to sponsor each of these goals. The board approves specific success measures for each goal, such as reducing outpatient waiting time from arrival to lab draw to 10 minutes with results reported to the MD within 1 hour for the patient's visit, or reducing outpatient x-ray waiting time to 10 minutes with results reported to the MD within 40 minutes (using digital x-ray). (I am aware of a very large clinic that consistently achieves both of these quality goals.) The senior executive sponsor forms a strategic goal team that meets monthly to review action plans and charter improvement projects (task forces) to achieve the board's objectives. Call these "board-approved strategic goal teams." The improvement project task forces report monthly back to the executive sponsor's strategic goal team, which redirects, approves/rejects recommendations, and makes resource allocations. The executive sponsor reports to the board quarterly on progress made by the strategic goal team and its task forces. Any task forces reporting to a strategic goal team are generally short-term do-it groups (DIGS). It's important to have a "sunset date" spelled out within the charter of each board-approved strategic goal team. As you might imagine, many projects and task forces may be initiated by the board-approved strategic goal teams. However, it still remains important to actively encourage proposals from a frontline rapid improvement team (RIT) and rapid improvement circles (RICs) of employees that report their results to the hospital's main quality and cost improvement council. (See steps 15 and 17.) It's very important to share all team charters among all the teams to avoid redundancy. To that end, the vice president of quality and cost should be an ad hoc member of the board, to be aware of all board-initiated strategic quality and cost improvement goals and their executive sponsors.

The diagram in Figure 3.2 (in step 7) illustrates the organizational structure for improving quality and cost and includes board-approved strategic goal teams. *It is critical to build such an ongoing quality and cost-improvement structure into the organizational structure, so that it continuously and automatically functions within the organization.*

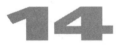

Publish an Annual Quality Report for Simultaneous Review with the Annual Financial Report

Publish an annual (or more frequent) quality report that the board and other stakeholders may view alongside the annual financial report. To make quality results continuously and easily accessible to the maximum number of employees, consider publishing them on your intranet. Also publish your quality and cost-improvement manual on the Internet for all to see. Certain approved people would have the ability to update it in real time on the intranet to continuously improve it into the future. Changes would be date stamped for reference. There should also be a brief printed booklet or brochure to explain quality system basics to employees and how to access the full quality system on the intranet. Because of the scope of developing and implementing a comprehensive quality management system, create a long-term "improvement team" of key stakeholders to help develop the quality-management system, so that they embrace it. Implementing a quality-management system on a corporate intranet provides the advantage that it allows the real-time viewing of current quality information, such as balanced scorecard information, related performance graphs, and statistical process control charts. As problems appear, corrective action is taken immediately.

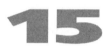

Create a Rapid Improvement Team to Make Quick Cost and Quality Improvements

Each member of the rapid improvement team (RIT) is to rapidly achieve and document significant cost and quality improvements at least monthly for a period of one to two years.

15.1 The RIT is composed of all department managers and/or supervisors in the organization. All areas are targeted for cost and quality improvement. The team meets biweekly or monthly. RIT members will later recruit frontline employees into improvement teams.

15.2 Give each RIT member a goal of reducing their budget by approximately 3 percent (to 10 percent) within a year. Alternatively, ask each team member to achieve a documented benchmark status of being in the top 25 percent of all comparable departments across the United States in terms of cost and quality. Each team member then documents a specific cost reduction/quality improvement on at least a biweekly or monthly basis until they achieve their goal. That is, they actually achieve an improvement, not just entertain an idea, every two weeks to a month. They each submit the improvements that were actually achieved to the RIT facilitator by completing a cost and quality improvement form. One rapid improvement team, which I facilitated a few years ago, achieved $3.5 million of cost reductions in six months, with a projected three-year savings of $14 million, without any layoffs. Comparable success can be achieved by any committed healthcare organization. A reasonable cost and quality improvement goal would be to achieve best 25th percentile benchmark status, or alternatively a dollar-cost reduction of approximately $4,000 per occupied bed per year. Benchmark values are available from companies such as VHA, Premier, Solucient, and Hewitt Associates. Don't spend excessive time creating and maintaining complex benchmarking systems. They tell you only where you've been. The only way to progress is to take action to improve processes. So, use simple benchmarks like comparing FTE's per adjusted patient day, or cost per CMI adjusted discharge. See the simple benchmarking chart for automakers that appears in Appendix A. You can similarly create a simple benchmark comparison among healthcare providers in your region. It's better to spend your time carefully observing and improving processes rather than maintaining complex benchmarking systems.

15.3 Form a parallel team to address the rising cost of prescription drugs and other advanced diagnostics and treatments (such as in radiology). This pharmacy and therapeutics team, like the RIT, should report directly to the hospital's main Quality and Cost Improvement Council, which will help set specific goals for both. A study performed by PricewaterhouseCoopers in 2002 found that 22 percent of rising costs in healthcare were due to the increase costs of prescription drugs and other advances in diagnostics and treatment. Yet, pharmaceutical companies spend huge sums on advertising campaigns for their products. Pharmaceutical costs are even more troubling, since Americans pay on average twice the amount paid for the same drugs as do the French and Italians. Similarly Americans pay 78 percent more than Swedes, 74 percent more than Germans, and 67 percent more than Canadians for the same drugs. This has led to a thriving practice of Americans buying their prescriptions in Canada. Rising drug and hospital costs are the two biggest causes of increasing healthcare costs; both must be addressed head on.

15.4   The rapid improvement team has a senior administrative leader (for example, a vice president or chief operating officer) who reports directly to the president/CEO. The RIT also has a facilitator/coordinator who can train team members in cost reduction and in process and quality improvement techniques. Given adequate knowledge, the senior administrative leader and the RIT facilitator may in fact be the same person. Alternatively, the RIT facilitator may be the head of the hospital's Cost and Quality Improvement Department or a designee. The point is that the RIT facilitator should report at a high level in the organization (for example, to the VP of Quality and Cost Improvement or to the CEO or COO) to illustrate the organization's commitment to improvement. The facilitator, all RIT members, plus the complete management team, the board, and all employees are visibly committed to rapid cost and quality improvement. One can't simply ask employees and physicians to shoulder extra improvement work without first building complete support from their bosses, that is, the board and all hospital administrators and managers.

15.5   The chair of the RIT (who may be the VP of Quality and Cost Improvement or Chief Operating Officer [COO]) should be a standing member of the hospital's main Quality and Cost Improvement Council, which reports to the board. The hospital's main Quality and Cost Improvement Council helps set major organizational goals for the RIT. The RIT facilitator may also be a member of the hospital's Quality and Cost Improvement Council. (See Figure 3.2 in step 7.)

15.6   The RIT facilitator also provides RIT members with continuing education at team meetings and may elicit the help of consultants having these skills. The facilitator and/or consultant teach team members a problem-solving methodology along with Toyota Lean Production methods. All VPs and the CEO are invited to selected RIT training sessions so that they too absorb the new improvement methods. There are many problem-solving methodologies. Table 3.1 presents basic problem-solving methodologies, while Table 3.2 presents improvement philosophies. Toyota Lean Production is an improvement philosophy or framework that is implemented around a problem-solving methodology. What's most important is not the particular improvement philosophy and problem-solving methodology selected but rather the simple commitment of the organization to demonstrably pursue continuous cost and quality-improvement as part of its ongoing mission and values. Still, it is important for the organization to endorse and publish its quality/cost improvement methodology and philosophy and to eventually train all employees to use it relentlessly.

The RIT meets biweekly for a year or two or until the members are no longer able to achieve significant cost and quality improvements. After a year, they should have already captured most of the low-hanging fruit, in terms of cost and quality improvement opportunities, that they can individually see. At some point they need to be reenergized to accomplish more with the help of their frontline employees.

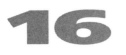 **Encourage RIT Members to Implement Toyota-Style Work Teams**

At Toyota each worker is called a "team member," since they work all day in teams of three to eight employees. All team members work near one another and are cross-trained to rotate to avoid repetitive

Table 3.1 Basic problem-solving methodologies.

I. Guided design	II. Plan, do, check, act	III. Focus PDCA	IV. Juran	V. Failure mode and effects analysis (FMEA)	VI. Six Sigma using DMAIC
1. Recognize problem.	1. Plan activities to improve a problem or process.	1. Find the process to improve.	1. Identify the problem.	1. Perform a detailed review of the product or process. Team may be used.	1. Define: Establish team and charter; identify sponsor and resources.
2. Define the problem.	2. Do— implement the improvement activities.	2. Organize (a team) to improve the process.	2. Establish the team.	2. Brainstorm all ways it can fail.	2. Measure: Confirm team goal; define current state; collect and display measures/data.
3. Identify alternative solutions.		3. Clarify understanding of the process.	3. Diagnose the cause.	3. List potential effects of each failure mode.	3. Analyze: Determine process capability and speed; determine sources of variation and time bottlenecks.
4. Consider consequences of major alternative solutions.	3. Check to see if the activities really do result in improvement.	4. Understand the root causes of variation in the results of the process.	4. Remedy the cause.	4. Assign 1 to 10 severity rating for each effect. 10 = high.	4. Improve: Generate ideas; conduct experiments; create straw models; develop action plans; implement.
5. Choose alternative for implementation, or rank the alternative solutions according to step 4.	4. Act—Either accept the final results or modify the plan in step 1 again and repeat the PDCA cycle.	5. Select the process improvement.	5. Hold the gains.	5. Assign 1 to 10 probability of occurrence rating for each failure mode. 10 = high probability.	5. Control: Develop control plan; monitor performance; mistake-proof process.
6. Implement the selected alternative.		6. Plan.	6. Replicate solution in other similar settings.	6. Assign 1 to 10 detection rating for each failure mode and/or effect. 10 = not detectable.	
7. Evaluate and control implementation.		7. Do.	7. Nominate new problems (i.e., return to step 1.)	7. Calculate risk priority number (RPN) for each effect. Severity # × Occurrence # × Detection #.	
8. Return to step 1 until desirable/optimal solution is obtained.		8. Check.		8. Prioritize failure modes for action via RPNs.	
Remark: In addition consider:		9. Act. Repeat PDCA steps 6 through 9 until a final solution is obtained. (PDCA described in prior column.)		9. Take action to eliminate/reduce the high RPN failure modes.	
A. Use team if desirable.				10 Calculate the resulting RPNs as the failure modes are reduced or eliminated.	
B. Resources available, as these may mean choosing a solution that may be second best.					
C. Constraints on the situation, as these may also mean choosing a solution that may be second best.					

Table 3.2 Improvement philosophies (that is, framework).

VII. Deming	VIII. Crosby	IX. Baldrige	X. ISO 9000	XI. Lean Toyota Production System
1. What are we doing and why, that is, state mission and values.	1. Management commitment.	1. Leadership.	1. Management responsibility.	1. Respect employees (mutual respect).
2. Improve quality.	2. Quality improvement team.	2. Strategic planning.	2. Quality system principles.	2. Permanent quality/cost improvement structure.
3. Cease dependence on mass inspection.	3. Quality measurement.	3. Customer and market focus.	3. Document control.	3. Cross-trained employee work teams.
4. Don't buy on price alone, but rather on how much you have to pay over the life of the product.	4. Calculate cost of quality.	4. Information and analysis.	4. Purchasing.	4. Improvement plan.
5. Constantly improve every process.	5. Quality awareness.	5. Human resource focus.	5. Identification and traceability.	5. Employee goals with strategic goals.
6. Train employees well using best-practice skills.	6. Corrective action.	6. Process management.	6. Control of processes and production.	6. Quality and cost improvement manual.
7. Show ethical leadership.	7. Zero-defect planning.	7. Business results.	7. Inspection and testing.	7. Continuous flow.
8. Replace fear with trust.	8. Supervisor training.		8. Nonconformance.	8. Visual workplace.
9. Remove barriers among staff areas. Cooperate throughout the organization so that all can win.	9. Zero defects day.		9. Corrective action.	9. Sequence and standardize work.
10. Eliminate slogans, exhortations, and arbitrary targets.	10. Goal setting.		10. Transport.	10. Quick changeovers.
11. Eliminate numerical quotas.	11. Error-cause removed.		11. Quality records.	11. Quality in station.
12. Remove barriers to pride and workmanship.	12. Recognition.		12. Internal audits.	12. Employees stop/fix defective processes.
13. Institute education and self-improvement.	13. Repeat from step 1 through 13.		13. Training.	13. Eliminate all waste: a. Overproduction. b. Poor staff utilization. c. Defects and rework. d. Waits and delays. e. Transportation. f. Unnecessary motion. g. Inventory. h. Overprocessing.
14. Accomplish a transformation to achieve the aim of the business.			14. Follow-up.	14. Help suppliers improve.
			15. Statistical techniques.	15. Hold all gains.
				16. Automate with ROI.

stress, add variety to their jobs, and cover for and help one another when needed. Creating an effective team is not always easy, as it means that the workers learn a wide variety of skills. In addition to multiple assembly functions, Toyota team members also do house-keeping, minor tool repair, and quality checking; they are multifunctional. Being multifunctional is very efficient in that it eliminates hand-offs. Finally, some of the team members have time periodically set aside for suggesting ways to improve processes.

Each team has a leader who is an hourly worker selected by management rather than elected by their coworkers. The team leaders provide team members with whatever they need to do their jobs safely and effectively. Refer to a team of three to eight workers and its leader as a "work team."

There is also a group leader (analogous to a hospital manager or supervisor) who works with a number of teams. A group leader might work with up to eight teams with a grand total of fewer than 60 employees. The group leader also works alongside the other team leaders and members. Each team leader will immediately help a team member solve a problem. If necessary, the group leader will join in, and if they can still not solve the problem they will all get together with the hourly and salary labor reps and work together in the Team Involvement office to quickly solve the problem.

Toyota uses this team and immediate problem-solving structure every day in its plants, and in particular in the Fremont, California, plant, which is called NUMMI for "New United Motor Manufacturing, Inc." The NUMMI plant was established in 1984 as a joint venture between Toyota and General Motors Corporation. NUMMI has helped change the U.S. automobile industry by introducing a team-based work environment as well as the Toyota Production System (TPS). The NUMMI facility was once solely a General Motors facility that had been described by one GM manager as the "worst plant in the world." In 1982, GM Fremont closed its doors. Toyota NUMMI began production at the old GM Fremont facility in 1984, with the same union leadership and with 85 percent of the workforce composed of former GM Fremont employees. Within two years, NUMMI was more productive than any other General Motors plant and had quality levels that rivaled those at its sister Toyota plant in Japan. If a failed U.S. automaker can remake itself using TPS into a world-class lean producer with highest quality, so too can any hospital, clinic, or health system. Today, NUMMI is a company with 5,440 team members who produce three award-winning vehicles: Toyota Corolla, Toyota Tacoma, and Pontiac Vibe. In 2002, NUMMI began producing the right-hand-drive Toyota Volz, which is exported to Japan. NUMMI has a collaborative partnership with the United Auto Workers and has five core values: teamwork, equity, involvement, mutual trust and respect, and safety. NUMMI was first to demonstrate the success of the Toyota teamwork system in the United States, and other U.S.-based Toyota plants have followed.[6]

Ask for volunteers among RIT members who wish to try the Toyota team approach in their departments. Certain large hospital departments are particularly amenable to using Toyota-style work teams to better organize daily work, such as surgical operating rooms, nursing units, emergency department, laboratory, radiology, pharmacy, physical therapy, medical records, word processing/transcription, food service, and human relations. The advantages of using the Toyota team structure include fast problem solving, task variety for workers sharing multiple jobs, flexibility of cross-trained workers to cover for one another, and built-in ongoing team contributions to continuous quality and cost improvement. The Toyota team structure is shown in Figure 3.5.

17 Implement Rapid Improvement Circles of Employees

After the rapid improvement team (RIT) loses energy and creative spirit in approximately a year, train each RIT member to carry cost reduction and quality improvement down to frontline employees in their departments. They may have already begun doing this by volunteering to implement Toyota-style work teams in their departments. Each RIT member is likely to be a department head or supervisor. In addition, train all RIT members to form quality and cost improvement circles in their departments from 4 to 12 months after the RIT is formed. These are different from the employee work teams, since they meet only weekly or biweekly. They are synony-

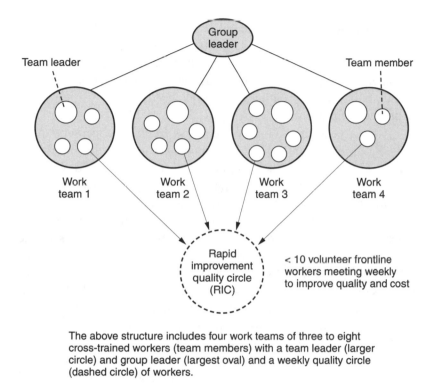

The above structure includes four work teams of three to eight cross-trained workers (team members) with a team leader (larger circle) and group leader (largest oval) and a weekly quality circle (dashed circle) of workers.

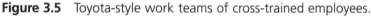

Figure 3.5 Toyota-style work teams of cross-trained employees.

mous with Toyota's quality circles. Toyota quality circles are improvement or self-improvement study groups composed of a small number of employees (10 or fewer) and their supervisor. The supervisor's role is likened to that of a coach and enabler, rather than of a boss. Quality circles originated in Japan, where they are called quality control circles. Quality circles are small groups of volunteer employees who meet on company time to identify, analyze, and solve local problems of their choice and present their solutions to management for implementation approval.

Train RIT members to teach and engage their employees within their new RIC quality and cost improvement circles. Use the name of "RIC" or "rapid improvement circle" for these circles of frontline employees. A current RIT member or a designee chairs each RIC. A key element is that each RIT member teaches his or her RIC members how to do continuous cost and quality improvement and then reports the results back to the RIT. Remember that the RIT is composed of all managers and supervisors of the organization, while each RIC is composed of 10 or fewer frontline employees meeting weekly or biweekly to propose improvements.

After a year, the RIT may meet less frequently, perhaps quarterly. RIT members may have implemented some Toyota-style work teams (Figure 3.5) in their departments to reorganize day-to-day operations. RIT members are now also chairing RIC quality circles and are learning more sophisticated improvement methods at now quarterly RIT meetings. The RIT helps set goals for the RICS, evaluates their progress, and reports successes and difficulties to the main quality and cost improvement council for the hospital. The weekly or biweekly RICs function as part of the organization's continuous quality and cost improvement effort, while the RIT continues to function as a reporting/training umbrella over the RICS. Employees working day to day in Toyota-style work teams also tend to support these efforts, since they feed suggestions to the RIC quality circles. The RIT or the RICs may also establish task forces designed to solve specific problems quickly, such as within 1 to 90 days. For that matter, any of the entities that appear in Figure 3.2 or Figure 3.5 may establish separate task forces reporting to them to solve specific quality and cost problems. Consider the name of "do-it group" (DIG) for any task force of 1 to 90 days that is directed at specific tasks.

A do-it group is essentially a kaizen improvement team charged with quickly improving a certain problem area. (Please also see improvement steps 30 and 31.) General Electric calls such kaizen improvement groups "work-out" groups, and they are charged with completing a significant improvement with a few days to a month. Other organizations sometimes refer to such quick improvements as Rapid Improvement Events (RIEs) or Rapid Process Improvements (RPIs). Each short-term task force would have a written charter containing its goals and sunset date. As a practical matter, it is wise to manage most task forces via either the RIT, which represent all managers and supervisors in the organization, or the RICs, which represent selected volunteer frontline employees. If other committees, teams, or short-term task forces are directed at quality and cost problems within the organization, it is important to have their charters available to all RIT members to avoid duplicating efforts.

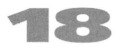 ## Implement a Permanent Organizational Structure for Quality and Cost Improvement

The structure shown in Figure 3.2 will continuously and permanently carry cost and quality improvement into the future with maximal use of internal staff and minimal expense. This structure is the most important element for the success of ongoing quality improvement and cost reduction. If a hospital can't afford expensive consultants or a large internal Quality and Cost Improvement department with numerous industrial engineers, then existing VPs, managers, supervisors, and employees can be trained to do quality and cost improvement within the structure of the internal RIT and its RICS and the board-approved strategic goal teams. All department mangers and frontline employees are champions of continuous quality improvement and cost reduction for the entire organization. New employees are quickly oriented to this system, so they can immediately make their contributions toward improvements.

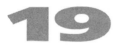 ## Set a Goal for Each RIC Member to Produce One to Four New Suggestions Per Month

Set a goal for each RIC member (frontline employee) to produce one to four new suggestions each month for cost and quality improvement after their first month of participation. Each RIC evaluates its department members' suggestions if not overly technical. Overly technical suggestions are referred to the Cost and Quality Improvement Department. In a high-performing RIC, according to Iwao Kobayashi in *20 Keys to Workplace Improvement,* "group objectives are almost always achieved through the efforts and desires of the members of the group. Everyone is achieving their personal desires while making significant improvement and enjoying each other's association in after-hours recreation." If a RIC loses energy, allow the RIC members to engage all the employees in their department by teaching them continuous quality improvement and cost reduction methods. The RIC may also invite new members from other departments so it becomes cross-functional, addressing problems among departments. Cross-functional teams are useful for solving difficult technical problems. Then extend the goal for every employee in the organization to make one or two new suggestions for cost or quality improvement each month. Go to work areas and ask employees what they can do at their workstation to make their job easier, and immediately record their suggestion on a suggestion form so they can receive credit. Then, do everything you can to make the suggester the implementer. And if implementation is beyond the worker's scope, make the worker part of the implementation team. Prioritize and implement the suggestions with the greatest cost benefit. Develop a reward system for employees whose suggestions have been implemented, whether the reward be hours of paid time off, award certificates, meal vouchers, sharing a percentage of the actual savings achieved, or a general gain-sharing program based on achieving annual profit and quality goals for the organization. If you have temporary or traveler employees, ask for their suggestions too and equally reward them. Remember, they may have worked for many other organizations and can share valuable suggestions. At Toyota's NUMMI plant, it is interesting to note that in 2000, 70 percent of employees participated in turning in approximately 18,000 suggestions, and over 90 percent of those were implemented! In the United States, Toyota employees each contribute about 36 suggestions per year, or about three per month. This has achieved millions in savings, and employees were rewarded with a payout. They also participated in a gain-sharing program based on company financial goals. Worldwide, the Toyota Corporation in-house suggestion scheme generates more than 2 million ideas a year. Over 95 percent of the workforce contributes suggestions. That works out to more than 30 suggestions per worker per year. The most remarkable statistic from Toyota is that over 90 percent of the suggestions are implemented worldwide. In Japan, the average Toyota employee contributes 329 improvement suggestions to the company each year, or more than one per workday.

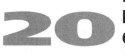

Have a Clear Reward and Recognition Program, and Communicate Negative Consequences

As has been mentioned, it's critical to motivate everyone to participate in cost and quality improvement. This means having a clear award/recognition system to recognize outstanding contributions and performance. It means having a reward system to share benefits with those contributing to positive results. This includes award/reward/recognition systems for physicians, practitioners, and other key stakeholders, as well as employees. Everyone needs to be involved and motivated. Develop a gain-sharing program for employees who meet organizational performance goals. This includes frontline employees as well as top administrators. The hospital's board of directors approves these award/reward/recognition and gain-sharing programs to support its strategic objectives. In addition, publish your positive results in newsletters and newspapers for all to see. Implement a good recognition system to publicly thank those contributing to your lean successes. Finally, be up front about any negative consequences that may occur if cost and quality improvement targets are missed.

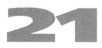

Adopt and Teach Continuous Improvement to as Many People as Possible in the Organization

Permanently embed continuous quality and cost improvement into the organization using Toyota Lean Production and a problem-solving methodology adopted from Table 3.1. Senior management would learn Toyota-style principles and the improvement methodology first, followed by the rapid improvement team members, then the rapid improvement circle members, and then as many employees as possible. Distribute the short, straightforward, easy-to-understand Quality and Cost Improvement Manual for quick reference throughout the organization. The main Quality and Cost Improvement Council approves this manual. Initially use the problem-solving method that best fits your organization's philosophy. It's not so important which method you first pick, but that you just pick one and begin. Personally, I recommend beginning with the guided design method within the Toyota Lean Production framework and later migrating to more complex problem-solving methods from Table 3.1. Guided design emphasizes the thorough consideration of all alternatives, and a slow and deliberate evaluation process followed by rapid decision and implementation. Invest the time needed with stakeholders to enroll them in the problem-solving process, and obtain their consensus for the chosen solution (*nemawashi*). Reflect on the shortcomings of improvement projects (*hansei*), and avoid those mistakes in the future.

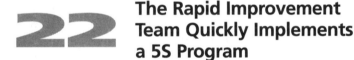

The Rapid Improvement Team Quickly Implements a 5S Program

The goal of a 5S program—sort, set in order, shine, standardize, and sustain—is to organize and clean all workplaces. It's good to have a rapid improvement team make a 5S "clean and organize" program as its first initiative. It takes about two weeks and demonstrates clearly visible, generally nonthreatening results. It is also a good way to get a quick success for RIT members. Each RIT member can use a digital camera to take before-and-after 5S pictures to show their dramatic successes. These pictures may be posted on two display boards entitled the "Wall of Fame," which was transformed from the old "Wall of Shame." This can be a fun way to illustrate 5S successes. Alternatively, use a before/after videotape to showcase especially dramatic successes. Complete the 5S program shown below in a short time, about 2 weeks:

> 1S—Sort. Remove all items from the workplace that aren't needed.

> 2S—Set in order. Arrange items so that they are easy to use, and label them so that they are easy to find and

put away. Arrange items to minimize transport time. Use shadow boards or floor outlines to clearly mark the correct locations for storing equipment. A certain area outlined on the floor with a painted stripe to hold a certain amount inventory, supplies, equipment, or work in process will immediately reveal any shortage or excess. To the extent possible, make all available equipment, instruments, and tools visible as opposed to putting them in closed or locked cabinets. To the extent possible, substitute open shelves and shadow boards for cabinets that hide things.

3S—Shine. Clean floors, shelves, counters, and equipment, and keep it that way daily. Maintain equipment frequently, starting with the most critical equipment first.

4S—Standardize. The first three S items are activities, while *standardize* is the method we use to continue all three of those activities continuously. Document the standard way of how and when the first three steps are done.

5S—Sustain. Make a habit of properly maintaining the standardized methods. If the staff does all the above steps but doesn't adopt the habit of doing so, all will revert to the way it was before.

A neat, clean, and organized facility has higher productivity, produces fewer errors and defects, meets schedules and deadlines better, and is a safer place to work. The following are examples of waste when a 5S program is ignored:

Excess inventory cost

Effort to continually rearrange excess inventory

Unneeded transport of items

Obsolescence of excess inventory

Quality defects from aging inventory

Equipment breakdowns from interfering dirt and debris

Unneeded equipment and inventory poses a daily obstacle to productive work

Unneeded items make designing smooth workflow difficult

Appendix C presents a real-life healthcare example of 5S as implemented at the VA Pittsburgh Healthcare System. Credit for this example goes to VA Pittsburgh Healthcare System's RN team leader, Ellesha McCray; CEO Michael Moreland; and Pittsburgh Regional Healthcare Initiative's communications director, Naida Grunden.[7]

The Pittsburgh Regional Healthcare Initiative (PRHI) is a consortium of the institutions and people who provide, purchase, insure, and support healthcare services in their region. Their partners include hundreds of clinicians, 42 hospitals, four major insurers, dozens of large- and small-business healthcare purchasers, corporate and civic leaders, and elected officials. Their goals are:

- Achieving the world's best patient outcomes by
- Creating a superior health system, by
- Identifying and solving problems at the point of care.

They are working to achieve perfect patient care in more than a dozen counties in the Pittsburgh area using the following patient-centered goals:

- Zero medication errors. More than 300 million medication errors occur every year in the United states, or about one per every U.S. resident.
- Zero healthcare-acquired (nosocomial) infections. About one in 14 hospitalized patients acquires an infection in the hospital.
- Perfect clinical outcomes, as measured by complications, readmissions, infections, and other patient outcomes, in:

    —Coronary artery bypass graft surgery.

    —Critical care and emergency medicine physicians.

    —Chronic conditions: depression and diabetes.

There is an excellent DVD video available from www.managementwisdom.com titled "How Hospitals Heal Themselves." It showcases the improvement efforts at PRHI and SSM Healthcare of St. Louis, MO. It includes an excellent companion book of improvement ideas titled "The Nun and the Bureaucrat" (2006).

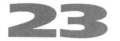

Identify Unnecessary Items Using Red Tags

Implement a red-tag holding area within each department, as well as a final red-tag holding area for the entire organization, to temporarily hold excess equipment and inventory that is in question. Make red tags to record item name, date tagged, number of items covered by the tag, reasons why the red tag is attached, department responsible for the item, the optional value of the item, and so forth. The best way to carry out red tagging is to do the whole target area quickly, in one or two days. In fact, many companies choose to complete the entire red-tagging process in one or two days for the entire company. At this stage, just tag the items in question without necessarily evaluating what you are going to do with them. After a limited time, such as two weeks, evaluate what you are going to do with each red-tagged item. Options are: keep it in the department or final red-tag holding area for further evaluation, move it to a new location in the work area, store the item away from the work area, or dispose of it (throw away, sell, donate, return to vendor, lend out, distribute to another part of company, or send to a final red-tag holding area). Make a logbook to show the disposition of all red-tagged items. Summarize the results and benefits of the red-tag effort. Often companies think they need to build more space when they may discover plenty of space by using a red-tag effort.

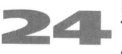

Promote Visual Control Throughout the Workplace and Organization

Visual control means "management by sight," that is, the actual progress of work is always visible. The concept of visual control may be physically extended in the sense of having all departmental work processes as visible as possible to any employee or observer. This means removing as many barriers as possible in departments to promote visibly efficient operation. Healthcare organizations generally use many managers, supervisors, and administrators, many of whom have private offices. Promoting visual control implies minimizing the number of private offices so that all work activities are visible and so that as many employees as possible, including mangers and administrators, are visibly doing value-added work that the patient would actually choose to pay for. This implies using more working supervisors and managers who actually share the value added work-load with their employees, in addition to managing. Certain private common areas may be reserved for confidential activities such as employee evaluations or rapid problem-solving sessions involving multiple participants. Reducing private office space may be a controversial initiative, but is consistent with the Toyota principle of visual control.

Visual control also means having inventory, supplies, instruments, and equipment visible to the workers. Closed cabinets, closed supply closets, and opaque enclosure are discouraged. Rather, everything should be visible and within easy reach and access.

Finally, it is also good to have key parameters of work processes visible. A simple control board (*andon*) can show at a glance the current work pace (*takt* time) and the location of any trouble. Takt time, or pace, is obtained by dividing the total time available per day by the required number to produce per day. So if a medical record area is supposed to process 160 records per 16-hour workday (two shifts), the takt time would be 960 minutes/160 records or 6 minutes per record. That's the needed pace to accomplish the effort. Kanban slips attached to supplies show how many are needed, where they came from, and where they are going. Standard worksheets visible at each work area show exactly how the process steps are to be performed. A standard worksheet describing the process steps will increase efficiency by displaying the workers' best production ideas and also prevent errors and accidents. This is all possible with an inconspicuous standard worksheet. The worksheet will typically contain the cycle time of process steps, the specific work sequence of the steps, and the standard inventory that will be used and produced. *Cycle time* is the time needed to carry out a sequence of steps to produce a given result. *Work sequence* refers to the to the order of operations that the employee carries out, such as transporting items, doing activity steps, and removing items, or moving them on to the next process. It does not refer to the order of all the processes, just the steps that concern the employee. It is the job of the supervisor to train the workers in the standard procedure. Standard worksheets must be simple, clear, and concise, and clearly visible to the involved employees.

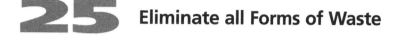 ## Eliminate all Forms of Waste

Recall our estimates that up to 50 percent of healthcare is essentially waste. Taiichi Ohno, the father of the Toyota Production system, stated, "Eliminating waste must be a business's first objective." The goal is to do only the actions that the patient will actually pay for and to consider everything else to be waste. Teach all employees (including RIT and RIC members) to identify waste as "gold, silver, or iron" according to the value of the waste, and then focus on removing or mining the waste that is "gold, then the silver, then the iron." In other words, go after the waste that is most "valuable" to the organization. In his book *20 Keys to Workplace Improvement* (page 155), Iwao Kobayashi says to post a "Treasure Mountain Map" in a central location to show workers where and to what extent waste exists in the workplace. This creates a friendly competition among workers to "mine the mountain of waste." This waste, or muda, is defined as any activity that adds cost but no customer value to a process. It can be categorized as follows:

25.1 Overproduction or Producing the Wrong Product Entirely

Providing products or services that aren't truly needed wastes resources that could be used to produce products or services that the customer really wants and needs (see Figure 3.6). Verify that the products or services you provide are indeed of highest value to patients. Recall that according to the *New England Journal of Medicine* study, patients typically receive only 55 percent of recommended care. Is the healthcare provider delivering the appropriate care to the patient in a cost-effective manner? I usually ask what the charge is for a medical procedure beforehand even though I have

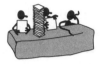

Producing more and/or faster than needed or producing the wrong product/service

Symptoms	Actual examples
• Not following care paths	• Patients typically receive 55% of recommended care
• Performing services patient doesn't need, for example, lab work	• 25% of surgical supplies picked and returned to shelf
• Unbalanced staff scheduling	• Picking OR instruments but not using them so they must be resterilized
• Having more than needed of anything, for example, beds	
• Extra floor space utilized	• Not notifying food service of diet changes and discharges
• Unbalanced material flow	• Repeatedly printing "face sheets" on nursing units
• Backups between departments	

Figure 3.6   Waste of overproduction.

insurance. I'm told by my friends that I'm rare in doing so. I'm usually surprised that the physician has only a vague idea of the charge to the patient. I have been surprised by responses like, "I'm a doctor; you'll have to ask the business office." It is wise to post the charges for common procedures and supplies for all physicians and nursing staff to see in their work areas. You'll probably get a reaction from them like, "I had no idea." With these patient charges visible every day, they may begin to use those services more cost effectively. They'll also be able to communicate costs better to patients, especially the uninsured.

25.2 Incorrect Utilization of Staff

This form of waste has three variations: (a) using the wrong level of staff for a certain task, (b) understaffing or overstaffing within the organization, and (c) not fully using an employee's skills and potential. I classify understaffing as a form of waste, as it will eventually lead to burnout and the loss of the employee if it is chronic. The wasted costs of rehiring and retraining then follow. Approximately 60 percent of total hospital costs are labor costs. In order to control healthcare costs, it's critical to control labor costs. This means having a responsive staffing system that accurately allocates staff to each work area based on numbers of patients (or procedures) and their acuity, that is, based on workload. If the workload in an area is excessive at any given time, it's critical to quickly move similarly qualified staff from less-used areas. Be responsive to shift to shift changes in workload. If the workload spikes up, add staff, but if it dips down remove staff. A pool of float staff can facilitate these moves. If the workload falls, you may schedule some staff to work on improvement teams and projects. Avoid fixed staffing levels that are not responsive to changing workload. To the extent possible, level out the workload by scheduling patients in a predictable manner, in accordance with the staff who are scheduled. If the patient scheduling system and the staffing scheduling system don't correspond to one another on a day-to-day and shift-to-shift basis, frequent problems will arise.

In order to be most cost efficient, it is critical that activities be performed by the lowest level of staff (that is, most frontline and lowest paid) who are qualified and skilled to perform the job. In addition, it's very important for any operational decisions to be made at the lowest possible level that is appropriate. Too often, operational changes that can produce immediate benefit are unnecessarily postponed for approval by some executive. It is often a waste of the executive's time, when the decision to implement an improvement could have been made at the level of the work team. It's sufficient for the work team to keep its group leader or manager apprised of improvements being made and to consult the leader on controversial changes. This speeds improvement and flattens the organization structure at the same time.

A good example of unnecessary waste is having numerous RNs doing certain operating room tasks that could be performed just as well by OR techs. Another specific example I observed was a full-time RN who was doing only repetitive phlebotomy (blood draws). A well-trained phlebotomist would have done the job just as well and more cost effectively. However, cross-training staff to perform multiple tasks is a good way to increase their value and versatility to help out whenever and wherever needed. The simple principles of cross-training staff to be more versatile and having the lowest level of qualified staff performing, managing, and improving tasks are not as rigorously practiced in healthcare as in Toyota Lean Production. How often do supervisors and managers assist with frontline healthcare activities?

How often do frontline healthcare staff rotate jobs with other team members? At Toyota, a team leader may lead a continuous improvement team but will also fill in for absent employees or whenever needed to solve immediate production problems. If healthcare workloads are too light and staff can't easily be moved to areas of greater need, then it's important to immediately offer them the option of time off without pay. The bottom line is that it's critical to achieve balanced and equitable staffing levels throughout a healthcare organization based on the workload present each shift and each day. A system to schedule, allocate, and redistribute staff based on continually changing workload remains a critical element for controlling healthcare costs. A computerized system to schedule and allocate staff may be good investment to reduce healthcare costs. Or can you develop a simpler nonautomated system to continuously and fairly allocate staff?

Gradually minimize job classifications among employees. This is an emotionally charged issue, but at least try to slowly move toward fewer job classifications. Excessive job classifications and specialization increases idle time, handoffs, and so forth. Consolidation of job classifications increases flexibility and thereby reduces those forms of waste. Interestingly, there are just three job classifications at the California NUMMI Toyota plant to set team members apart: production, tool and die, and general maintenance worker. This compares to dozens of job classifications at most other U.S. automakers. Team members routinely rotate jobs within their small teams. Multifunctional workers eliminate handoffs.

25.3 Defects and Rework

Defect examples include medication errors, incorrect surgeries, and poor clinical outcomes. Rework examples include retesting, rescheduling, resubmitting lost or rejected insurance claims, rewriting patient demographics, and multiple bed transfers. All represent unnecessary effort and wasted resources, and they contribute to ongoing quality problems. Any type of inspection well after an original process may also be considered rework. All checking is waste and may be prevented by error-proofing the original process. Create a culture to fix the cause of problems as they are encountered (that is, *jidoka* or quality in station). Build a visual system to quickly show problems when they arise, so they can be immediately fixed. Avoid using a computer screen if it pulls the employee away from doing value-added work. Allow any employee to "pull the cord" to "stop the process" and immediately fix it. Future occurrences are then minimized. This is what happens in a Toyota plant with simple andon lights signaling the problem on the stopped assembly line. (*Andon* is the Japanese word for paper lantern.) An andon board (Figure 3.7) lets supervisors know the location of the problem with a blinking light and a distinct musical tone.

Any employee can stop the line to resolve a problem. "Processes producing 'just in time' do not need extra inventory. So, if a prior

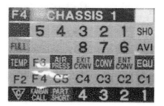

Figure 3.7a   Andon board.

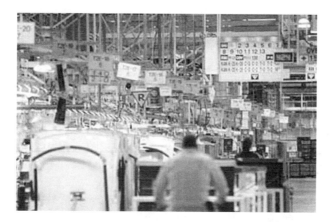

Figure 3.7b   This lighted board shows where an andon cord has been pulled to signal a problem on the line at Toyota Motor Corp.'s plant in Georgetown, Kentucky. If the issue is not fixed before the car reaches the next stage of assembly, the line stops.

process step generates defective parts, the next process step must stop the line. This makes defects immediately apparent. Furthermore, everyone sees when this happens and the defective part is returned to the earlier process. It is an embarrassing situation meant to help prevent the recurrence of such defects."[8] Toyota uses a green andon light to show all is normal, yellow to show that a worker is adjusting something, and red to show that a worker has stopped the line to rectify a problem. A new production line may stop frequently as problems are resolved but then begin to run smoothly, continuously, and efficiently. Ultimately, the number of errors will fall, and the line will almost never stop. Today in Toyota plants, where every worker can stop the line, it almost never stops and yields approach 100 percent. Toyota encourages employees to pull the cord, despite the line stoppages, to expose problems and address them quickly. In Toyota's plant in Georgetown, Kentucky, workers pull the "line stop" cords 2500 times a shift to signal problems, but actual stoppages amount to six to eight minutes per shift.[9] Yasuhiro Monden, author of a manual used at Toyota's California NUMMI plant, writes of the assembly line, "It is not a conveyor that operates men; it is men that operate a conveyor."

One may not see lighted boards near the ceilings in hospitals or clinics flashing problems. But in healthcare, it's easy for any employee to similarly "stop a defective process" with a simple explanation to the other team members and a page or phone call to the supervisor, team leader, or manager. At that time they can all ask "why" five times to determine the true root cause of the problem and correct it so that it will never happen again. Unfortunately, this mentality of immediately identifying a problem and permanently eliminating it isn't common enough in healthcare. Even though Toyota-style andon boards aren't often seen in hospitals, they could be considered in high production areas like operating rooms, supply processing, emergency departments, and nursing units.

Quickly fixing problems as they occur involves having a support system that can quickly put solutions in place. The idea is to resolve the problem as soon as it crops up. Toyota employees all work in teams of three to eight members and are generally referred to as team members. Each team has a team leader who is selected rather than elected. The team leader is there to provide team members with whatever they need to do their jobs safely and effectively. The team leader does the same work as the other team members, but he or she also coordinates the team, and in particular, fills in for any absent workers, an uncommon concept in U.S. mass production. A group leader over a number of teams also works alongside the team leaders and members.

When someone pulls the andon cord to signal a problem, the team leader may immediately help solve the problem. It is not uncommon to also see maintenance workers picking up production tasks to help with the problem. If necessary the group leader will join in, and if they still cannot solve the problem they will get together with the hourly and salary labor reps to all work side by side in the team involvement office to solve the problem. Taiichi Ohno stated that companies should have a system that immediately responds to a problem when it occurs. This is a marked contrast to historical American mass production, in which the assembly line was virtually never stopped and problems were fixed after automobiles rolled off the end of the line or, even worse, after the customer took possession. At the Toyota NUMMI plant, team members are also each given a "personal touch fund of $15" so that they can meet off hours to further solve problems. Now many American companies are embracing lean to reduce costs even though it may involve wrenching changes. This is a necessity if U.S. producers are to respond to worldwide competition from low-cost countries such as China and Mexico. These companies are now pushing to have healthcare providers adopt similar approaches to reduce skyrocketing healthcare costs, which are a major expense for them.[10] To avoid conflicts in adopting these approaches within healthcare, it's important to be sensitive to perceived differences in the "culture of caring healthcare" compared to the "culture of manufacturing efficiency." It may take years to fully transfer Toyota lean production methods to certain areas of healthcare, but targeting to begin to do so in months rather than years is advised. There will be starts, stumbles, stops, and even back steps along the way, but improving processes is the key to improving healthcare quality and costs.

Wherever possible, Toyota uses machines that stop themselves if defects are detected (jidoka or autonomation). They also require workers to stop the line if they detect any defect or abnormal condition. The jidoka (quality in station) philosophy shows faith in the team member as a thinker and allows all team members the right to stop the line on which they are working. Jidoka prevents defects from continuing, and allows the situation to be immediately investigated and corrected. The idea is to build in quality by preventing any defect from going to the next process. Each worker is an inspector for his or her own work and that of coworkers. This results in a working system that is designed to provide highest quality and lowest cost with minimal inspection.

It is important to mistake-proof (poka-yoke) processes whereever possible. Poka-yoke essentially makes it impossible for a particular defect to occur. Literally translated, the Japanese word *yokeru* means "to avoid," and *poka* means "unintentional error." So *poka-yoke* is translated as "avoiding unintentional errors." An everyday-life example is a buzzer going off in your car if you open the door with your headlights on. This is a detection poka-yoke that alerts the operator of an error to prevent a defect, such as the battery going dead. A prevention poka-yoke would be having the unleaded gas pump nozzle smaller so that it will only fit in the smaller gas tank insert. This prevents the error from ever occurring. Think about it. Every time you put gas in your car, you are in fact automatically inspecting that you are using unleaded gas based on the size of the pump nozzle. Another prevention poka-yoke is not allowing a car to start unless the shifter is in the "park" position. A healthcare poka-yoke may mean storing no lethal or harmful doses of drugs anywhere, particularly on nursing units, to prevent an overdose. It may mean having equipment that can be connected only in the recommended manner, thus avoiding potential injury. It may mean having buzzers on equipment to signal dangerous conditions. It may mean automatically isolating certain infected patients in a manner to prevent the spread of the infection. It may also mean always using disposables to prevent spread of infection.

Perform root-cause analyses to eliminate the causes of defects and rework and implement countermeasures. Like Toyota workers, ask "why" five times to get at the real cause of the problem. Analyze and/ or try alternatives until the problem is resolved. Maintain a continuous improvement program to minimize defects/rework. Continuously aim to reduce defects to zero.

Six Sigma is a quality improvement methodology that follows the DMAIC steps of define, measure, analyze, improve, and control, and its goal is to reduce process variation and eliminate defects.

| Inspect and/or repair a defective service or product |

Symptoms	Actual examples
• Adverse drug events	• UR, infection control, legal, and risk management inspections
• High infection rates and falls	
• High incidence of bill rejects	• Lack of standardized script at registration
• Frequent rescheduling of office appointments	
• Multiple quality control checks	• Replacing "lost" gowns in OR/nursing
• Patient returns (OR, readmit)	• Inappropriate communication of patient transfer mode with order entry
• Missed shipment/deliveries	
	• Pharmacy refilling "multiple dose" medications

Figure 3.8   Waste of correction.

Fortune 500 companies like GE, Motorola, and McKesson implement Six Sigma programs to reduce defect rates to less than 3.4 per 1,000,000. Six Sigma improvements are driven by data. Six Sigma focuses on projects that will produce measurable business results. Using Six Sigma, GE Capital saved $2 billion in 1999. There is nothing magical about Six Sigma, and it shares much with other past improvement methods. The "define" step presents a clear explanation of the problem/project. The "measure" step illustrates how much variation there is in the process. The "analyze" step looks at alternatives to improve the process and reduce variation and defects to Six Sigma targets. The "improve" step implements those changes. Finally, the "control" step ensures that the newly improved processes will not revert to prior excess variability and defect levels. Six Sigma is based upon improving processes by understanding and controlling variation, thus improving the predictability of results. So, study the variation in processes and their defect rates, and systematically minimize both. (See Figure 3.8).

25.4 Waits and Delays

Organize the work so that there are as few delays as possible. Examples are waiting for medical appointments, medical assessments,

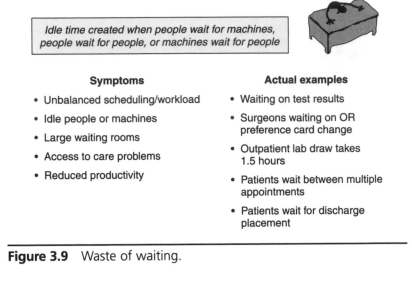

Idle time created when people wait for machines, people wait for people, or machines wait for people

Symptoms	Actual examples
• Unbalanced scheduling/workload	• Waiting on test results
• Idle people or machines	• Surgeons waiting on OR preference card change
• Large waiting rooms	• Outpatient lab draw takes 1.5 hours
• Access to care problems	• Patients wait between multiple appointments
• Reduced productivity	• Patients wait for discharge placement

Figure 3.9   Waste of waiting.

ancillary tests to be performed, test results, bed assignments, surgical and nonsurgical scheduling, presurgical testing, OR prep, and payment cycle times. Unnecessarily monitoring patients or watching equipment operate is another example of waste. When possible, do intermediate steps in parallel at the same time. Study each step and sub process and reduce its length of time. (See Figure 3.9.)

25.5 Transportation

The act of moving materials or information around clearly doesn't add any value to the customer or patient. Actually, any transport process in itself is non-value added and needs to be eliminated or at least minimized. (See Figure 3.10.)

25.6 Unnecessary Motion

People and equipment are rarely where they are needed. A past example is requiring a patient to see a primary-care provider before seeing a specialist who is clearly needed. Searching for things and restacking inventory are other examples from the waste of unnecessary motion (see Figure 3.11). Employees stretching and walking to reach materials represents non-value-added procedures and waste.

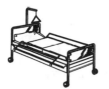

Any material or information movement

Symptoms

- Inappropriate bed assignments on admission

- Having multiple information systems

- Excessive medical records pickups and deliveries

- Extra hand-offs of anything

Actual examples

- Temporary warehouses and multiple storage locations

- Walking intermittent samples to lab and going to get prescriptions

- Staff copies patient chart for transfer between facilities

- Finished ED patient chart walked to financial counselor

- Multiple copies of surgery schedule distributed daily

- Every outpatient visit requires driver's license

Figure 3.10   Waste of transport of material and information.

Any movement of people or equipment

Symptoms

- Excess patient transfer/movement

- Convoluted facility and workplace layouts

- Prolonged pre-op test times

- Inconsistent work methods

- Reduced productivity

- Long reach/walk distances

- Long leadtimes for anything

Examples

- Walking intermittent samples to lab and going to get prescriptions or supplies

- Searching for anything, e.g., equipment

- ED triage, registration, treatment room, x-ray, financial counselor

- Poor workplace layout for patient services

- Locations of fax/copy machines

Figure 3.11   Waste of unnecessary motion.

Equipment may be difficult to prepare, load, and clean. Regardless of how much a worker moves, it does not mean they have completed meaningful work (move ≠ work). An employee may keep busy for hours just looking for things and never accomplish any meaningful work. He or she is just adding to the cost and lengthening the service time. All needed supplies and equipment should be near the worker. Walking adds no value. Accomplishing meaningful work means that the worker has completed value-added steps efficiently and with as little motion as possible. Use 5S to standardize, minimize, and organize work environments.

25.7 Excess Inventory

Minimize the amount of preprocess inventory, in-process inventory, and end-of-process inventory. Set a goal to reduce the total of all inventory in the organization by 50 percent or more (Figure 3.12). Do not purchase supplies in large lots. Inventory, storage, and handling savings will more than offset savings achieved through volume discounts. Use two containers to hold supplies and inventory at the point of use. The second full container is there as your safety supply. When one is emptied, simply send it back to be refilled. The second full container is still there as your safety supply. Size the containers

Any supply in excess of just-in-time customer requirements for goods or services

Symptoms	Actual examples
• Multiple forms, multiple copies, multiple weeks' supplies	• Duplication of supplies in temporary storage areas, patient rooms, closets, etc.
• No standardization of supplies	
• Unused appointment slots	• ED filled dumpster from one outdated storage area
• Empty beds	• Surgical services—one cart alone had $250K of sutures
• Complex tracking systems	
• Multiple storage and handling	• Excessive duplication in OR, SPD, pharmacy, nursing units
• Extra rework/hidden problems	

Figure 3.12 Waste of inventory.

so there are no inventory/stock-outs. This system is simple, requires no costly automation, and minimizes the inventory at each site of use. This is called a kanban system, which Taiichi Ohno of Toyota invented in the 1950s. "He dictated that parts would only be produced at each previous step to satisfy the immediate demand of the next manufacturing step. As each container carrying parts was used up at a manufacturing step, it was sent back to the previous step, and this became the automatic signal for more parts."[11] This simple idea is enormously powerful and eliminates nearly all excess in-process inventories.

Alternatively, use a kanban ordering card to pull just the right amount of inventory to the next process step at the time it is truly needed. Kanban cards signal the need for more inventory at the right time and place. This can all be done without complex computer systems.

Minimize all inventories but maintain safe levels. Savings generated by reducing inventories and supplies will fall directly to the bottom line and immediately increase profits. Imagine the entire organization moving supplies on a series of intersecting, continuously moving conveyor belts. Each conveyor feeds supplies to each work process at the rate of supply consumption for that process, and no more. Only when supplies are depleted to minimum safety levels are those supplies replenished in minimum-order quantities. Replenishment is initiated only by actual consumption. Try to achieve process steps that require no inventory. After improvement, have employees eliminate any exposed inventory. Many areas in hospitals can take advantage of kanban systems to mtinimize inventory including central stores, SPD, pharmacy, food service, nursing units, and operating rooms—virtually any area with inventory. Start with the areas that contain the greatest dollar value of inventories.

A hospital materials manager once boasted to me that he was achieving "26 inventory turns a year." That means at any given time, the hospital had about two weeks of inventory on hand. In comparison, Toyota typically has an inventory of two hours of parts on hand, which equates to roughly 2500 inventory turns a year, or 100 times more efficient that the hospital materials manager's use of inventory. In his book *The Machine That Changed the World*, James Womack presents a chart that shows Toyota having two hours of parts inventory on hand versus two weeks at a General Motors plant in 1986.

General Motors, like the hospital materials manager, might also have boasted at that time about its inventory efficiency. Yet, Toyota was 100 times more efficient at minimizing its inventory.

I am aware of hospitals that achieve as little two inventory turns a year. That means they may keep as much as six months of supplies in inventory. Some hospitals consider six turns a year acceptable, which equates to two months of inventory. Retaining this much inventory simply increases cost. Many hospitals try to achieve a national target of 12 to 15 turns a year, while some consider 26 turns a great achievement. Every hospital should continuously strive to reduce inventories to safe but minimum levels.

Another example of Toyota's use of lean inventories is illustrated by the West Coast dock strike of September 2002. At that time a Toyota plant manager from Fremont, California, appeared on CNN, saying that his plant only had a day or two of Toyota engines and transmissions on hand even though these were shipped from Japan! Why is it that a Toyota assembly plant in California can operate with only a day or two of critical engines and transmissions from Japan, while a hospital in the United States needs two weeks of inventory principally made in the United States? It is now a challenge for hospital materials managers to safely minimize inventories and have those savings go directly to the hospital's bottom line. A goal of reducing hospital inventories by half by using kanban systems is reasonable, as demonstrated by Toyota and other lean producers. Note also that a kanban system is primarily a simple manual system without the need for staff to enter supply orders into sophisticated computer systems.

Use a kanban system to eliminate all the cost and overhead associated with costly, computerized order entry systems. The term *kanban* is usually defined piece of paper divided into three categories that is in a rectangular vinyl envelope. This information may also appear on the corresponding container:

Pickup information

Transfer information

Production information

At a glance, a kanban may also provide production quantity, time, method, sequence or transfer quantity, transfer time, destination, storage point, transfer equipment, and container.[12] The first rule of kanban is that the later process goes to the earlier process to pick up items. This reverses the conventional flow of production, transfer, and delivery. The later process must instead take what it requires from the earlier process when it is needed. This sets the pace for the earlier process.

In addition to reducing "in process" inventory with kanbans, it's important to reduce the amount of preprocess inventory. I'm aware of one large nonprofit system of 14 hospitals that has reduced the number of items in its inventory catalog from 250,000 to 70,000 through standardization and value analysis of supplies and equipment. It has reduced its catalog by over 70 percent and certainly has achieved great savings in the process. It intends to have a final catalog of 35,000 items, which amounts to an 85 percent reduction. That was a target suggested by DeLoitte and Touche consultants. When undertaking such a preprocess inventory reduction, it's wise to create a systemwide value-analysis team with membership from all facilities. This team would have a similar goal of reducing preprocess inventory by 80 percent and in-process inventory by 50 percent. Remember that these savings will fall immediately to the bottom line and essentially represent profit on the income statement.

Excess inventory just hides a multitude of underlying problems. Suzaki states, "Excess Inventory is the root of all evil."[13] Companies want to reduce the inventory and simultaneously expose and correct the underlying problems, such as:

Poor scheduling

Communication problems

Production imbalance between departments

Long setup times

Long transportation

Vendor deliveries

Equipment/instrument breakdown

Quality problems

Absenteeism

Lack of housekeeping and organization

25.8 Excess Processing

Extra unneeded steps are often used to achieve a result. "Over-processing" represents waste. Complex registration processes are common examples of excess processing in healthcare (Figure 3.13). I have seen returning laboratory outpatients go through a very time-consuming, full hospital registration process before having their blood drawn at one hospital, while outpatients at another hospital provide just their name, date of birth, home address, and confirmation of their insurance carrier. Another example of excess processing is multiple registrations, in which the patient is asked repeatedly for the same information. Excessive paperwork and entering duplicate information on computer screens are other examples. If a person records information once, there is no need to record it again if systems and forms are well designed. Toyota also tries to build a kind of "human intelligence" into its machines. A worker starting a task on one of these machines does not have to idly watch the machine do its job. He or she can instead do another

> *Effort that adds no value to the product or service from the customer's perspective*

Symptoms	**Actual examples**
• Asking the patient the same questions multiple times	• Duplicating physical assessment at triage and in treatment area
• Multiple signature requirements	• Placing OR scheduling information in multiple systems
• Extra copies of forms	• Punching holes in paper to place in patient chart
• Duplicate information system entries	• Idly watching equipment operate
• Distribution of reports	
• Longer lead time	
• Reduced productivity	
• Sorting, testing, and inspection	

Figure 3.13   Waste of excess processing.

productive task. There are probably examples of staff in healthcare watching a machine, task, process, or patient when careful design could eliminate the need for watching (continuous inspection). Designs to remove continuous inspection have to be implemented carefully so as to improve quality rather than degrade it. These designs may be most successful with equipment; that is, try to obtain equipment that works so well that there is no need to watch it. Such equipment will immediately and appropriately signal you if there is a problem.

Many types of meetings are also good examples of waste. For example, calculate the expense of a meeting in terms of the total staff, their hourly salaries, the total time consumed, and travel time. Always ask ahead of time, "What are the goals of the meeting?" and ask afterward if they were accomplished expeditiously. Always have a written agenda stating the meeting goals and agenda items with times and responsibilities allotted for each. Distribute the agenda at least two days ahead of time. The purpose of the agenda is to let members know exactly why they are coming and what will be expected of them. Use a simple one-page form to record the meeting's minutes and results that can be distributed within a day after the meeting. Always ask, "Is this meeting something the patient would pay for, or does most of it represent a kind of 'overprocessing waste' that a patient would not wish to pay for?" Similarly, multiple committees within an organization may have overlapping responsibilities. For every committee and task force, it's important to have a written charter defining goals and responsibilities. See the example charter in Figure 3.14. The charter for a task force should include a sunset date, after which the task force will no longer meet. A task force is generally considered to be a short-term work group to accomplish specific tasks within a limited time, from a few days to 90 days. Standing committees may be a permanent part of the organization with no sunset date. Other nonstanding committees may have multiple goals and a sunset date for accomplishing those goals. Task forces may report to committees. It is important to streamline the overall committee structure to eliminate overlap wherever possible and to choose the membership carefully to appropriately use all members. Any underused member can be an ad hoc member to be included only when necessary.

Sample Team Charter

Specific challenge (purpose):

Team leader/facilitator:

Executive sponsors:

Core team members:

Recorder:

Primary customer:

Tentative meeting schedule:

Sunset date:

Objectives and goals:

Key questions to answer:

Key activities:

Flowcharts to compose:

Figure 3.14 Sample team charter.

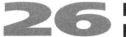 **Reduce Specific Examples of Potential Waste**

There is much potential for the elimination of waste in healthcare. As a preface to this paragraph, we should again all realize that a patient's healthcare is primarily delivered by the physician and nurse(s) and by supporting ancillary departments like lab, pharmacy, x-ray, and surgery, which provide tests, drugs, therapies, and interventions.

If a lean healthcare provider delivered best quality, many of the activities and positions below would be less needed. The following list is likely only a fraction of what might decrease in a truly lean, highest-quality healthcare organization. Remember Dr. Don Berwick's estimate that 40 percent of healthcare is waste, and Jim Womack's estimate that a truly lean organization can reduce labor, space, and inventory by half. It is a challenge for each healthcare provider and each of the following departments to embark on a lean journey of continuous cost and quality improvement to reduce the need for their own services. Just as it is said that a good consultant job is "to make his or her services no longer needed," so too it should be the goal in each of these and possibly other departments to reduce the need for their services by instead improving quality. The organization's principle of "respect for the employee" would ensure that each well-performing employee would still have a job for which he or she is qualified. Each of these employees is most likely a good, highly skilled, dedicated worker whose services may be redeployed elsewhere. Here are some examples of activities and positions that may be reduced if the highest quality were built into lean healthcare processes.

26.1 Excessive Layers of Administrators, Managers, Supervisors, and Inspectors

Scrutinize the numbers of administrators, managers, supervisors, and inspectors. As a challenge, ask your human resources (HR) department to count the number of "direct patient value-added employees," that is, the ones who directly service patients and for whom patients are totally willing to pay. HR may use a patient focus group if there are any doubts about a function being "patient value added." In 2000, a hospital HR consulting firm suggested an average target ratio of 16 employees per manager or supervisor when computed across the organization. Obviously some departments have many more employees per manager while others have much fewer. It would be good to obtain a new benchmark of this ratio in healthcare at this time. For contrast, I recall that Jack Welch targeted an average ratio of 25 to 30 employees per supervisor during his tenure at General Electric.

Then, compute the ratio of "direct patient value-added employees" divided by "total employees." You may find this percentage astounding. In addition, ask HR to compute total salary dollars for the direct patient value-added employees. Then divide that by the total salary dollars for all employees. You may be even more astounded by that percentage. It is an ongoing challenge to continually increase those two percentages.

26.2 Utilization Review Staff and Discharge Planners

This may be a big example of waste due to inspection. If proper utilization and discharge planning were built into existing patient-care processes, then most utilization review positions would go away. Basically, utilization review staffs continually recheck what physicians and nurses are doing, so that the patient leaves the hospital in a timely manner so that Medicare/Medicaid reimbursement will be sufficient. Insurance companies may also require utilization review staff to minimize the length of stay to match reimbursement. One large hospital where I once worked had about 40 such utilization review staff, most of whom were nurses who could be potentially providing direct care to patients.

26.3 Patient Advocate

A patient advocate is a hospital employee who receives patient complaints and then tries to satisfy the angry patient or passes the complaint on to someone who will prevent a recurrence. In an ideal healthcare delivery system, there would be little need for patient advocates as complaints would be minimal to nonexistent. The patient advocate position is symbolic for "rework in a patient process gone wrong."

26.4 Infection Control Nurses and Staff

If ideal sterile techniques were followed, there would be few infections and little need for these infection surveillance staff. A large hospital may have five such staff in a department. These staff monitor and report infections and help educate patient-care providers on how to best prevent infections. Not only is there cost associated with these surveillance staff, but there also is a far greater cost associated with the consequences of infections to patients. These consequential costs stem from extended lengths of patient stay, the use of specialized drugs, possible isolation, and follow-up interventions. One system of hospitals with a total of 885 beds estimated the consequential costs of infections at over a million dollars per year, not counting the cost of the infection surveillance staff themselves. In a truly lean, highest-quality hospital these staff would be completely focused on education to avoid all future infections. In the *Boston Globe Magazine,* Dr. Don Berwick states that if hospitals would impose a zero-tolerance policy for workers failing to wash their hands, that simple step could save more than 10,000 lives a year.[14] In fact, one in every 14 Americans admitted to a hospital receives an infection in the hospital. During my extended career in healthcare, on several occasions I have seen physicians use the men's room before beginning rounds and not wash their hands before leaving the men's room. Maybe it's time to have a sign above the sink or restroom door that says, "Please wash your hands before leaving." Use the Toyota principle of immediately responding to every infection (that is, defect) as it occurs to prevent all similar recurrences. Quickly and permanently eliminate identified root causes of infections, and then focus the infection control staff on continued educational efforts to "hold the gains." Some hospital CEO's have resorted to asking that every hospital acquired infection be immediately reported to them with an immediate actions to prevent future recurrence.

26.5 Managers, Supervisors, and Coordinators

If managers, supervisors, and coordinators don't provide direct patient care, are patients usually willing to pay for their services? If care processes were better designed, could these non-care-providing positions be reduced? Could they be converted to provide direct patient care?

26.6 Medicare Compliance Officer and Staff

A Medicare compliance officer is an on-staff "inspector" to ensure that Medicare regulations are being met. Because of past oversights, it is now a federal requirement to have a Medicare compliance officer. If Medicare regulations were continuously met in a high quality/ high-trust organization, these positions would not be necessary. They have come into vogue within recent years.

26.7 Legal Counsel for Patient Lawsuits

If highest-quality care and outstanding customer service were consistently provided, there wouldn't be any patient lawsuits and little need for these supporting attorneys. By contrast many hospitals employ several on-staff attorneys.

26.8 Safety/Risk Managers and Staff

Like lawyers, staff in this department are there to respond to major problems that may lead to patient litigation. If quality were built in, there would be no need for this function.

26.9 Marketing

Individual healthcare providers may spend hundreds of thousands of dollars annually marketing themselves via mailings, TV ads, and so forth. Is this something patients and their employers would choose to pay for? Why is so much advertising needed in healthcare? If we had a national system to equitably distribute healthcare resources, healthcare providers would not need to use advertising to compete for patients.

26.10 Numerous Financial Analysts/Auditors

Auditors essentially watch over all the department managers and how they budget and expend funds. One large three-hospital system with which I'm familiar had 22 such analysts. Why so many inspectors? If good financial management were built into departments, that number could be significantly reduced.

26.11 Excess Secretaries

Generally, the CEO and each vice president have a private secretary, and most department heads also have private secretaries. Why so many? A much smaller pool of secretaries that is shared by all would be much more efficient, for example, if it were located within a centralized transcription service and secretarial pool. Or, having one secretary shared among three or more vice presidents or department heads would be much more efficient. Healthcare providers have spent large sums in the past 20 years on personal computers, networks, and software to make communications and secretarial work easier. So, isn't it reasonable to share each secretary among three or more administrators and department heads? Remember that each department head now also has his or her own personal computer to help manage information and schedules.

26.12 Excess Information Technology

Hospitals and healthcare systems spend large sums on information technology without a clear return on investment. It appears to those providers that new and better information technology is just the right thing to do without clearly identifying cost and quality benefits. It's now time for every information technology purchase to have a clear return on investment analysis attached to it. If it doesn't provide a financial payback of less than so many years or achieve measurable quality improvement goals, it should be questioned. Is that purchase adding true value for the patient? Would an uninsured patient be willing to pay for this new technology? Purchasing more and more computer technology requires hiring more highly paid technical workers to maintain it, which detracts from its cost benefit. Lean value-added processes must come before adding more computer technology and automation. Still, if the new computer technology produces a truly desirable ROI and enables an organization to reach its quality goals, it's desirable after processes have first been improved.

It's now nearly standard for a personal computer to be on every desk, just like a phone, and to have a local area network connection, if not an Internet connection. There is enough computing power in each hospital to launch a mission to Mars. Each hospital now has a sophisticated Web site. Ask your information systems director how many hits each part of the hospital's Web site gets per month. You may be surprised by the low use of parts of your Web site that cost you so dearly. Also, how fast and responsive is your Web site? Do users exit the site because it's just too slow? Would patients have willingly paid for its development? Is the Web site directly benefiting patients and employees, or could those expenditures have been more prudently deployed? Some Web contents, such as job openings, clearly add value. Could your Web site have been more Spartan, providing just value-added information for patients and employees?

Speaking of Internet connections and e-mail, it is important that they be used appropriately for business purposes within an organization. Any company who thinks it's immune to Internet abuse should take note of these survey statistics from the *Technology Law Newsletter:*[15]

37 percent of employees surf the Web constantly at work.

8 percent of employees use workplace e-mail for personal use.

46 percent of online holiday shoppers make their purchases from work.

A recent audit of IRS employee usage of the Internet found that activities such as personal e-mail, online chats, shopping, and checking personal finances and stocks accounted for 51 percent of employees' time spent online! That's 51 percent of online time that people were supposed to have been doing value-added work! What percentage of time do employees spend online at your organization doing non-value-added activities?

Commercially available software can restrict personal Internet, chat, and e-mail usage.[16] Based on the above statistics usage monitoring software would appear to be a good investment for any company, including hospitals and clinics. Internet and e-mail abuse is another example of significant waste that is growing, and most providers aren't addressing it.

26.13 Government Relations

Some large hospitals/clinics have high-level government relations specialists on staff to study and help steer pending legislation. This is a type of overproduction. Again, it is not something most patients wish to pay for. What we need instead is a logical, national health-care strategy designed to increase quality and reduce cost.

27 Sequence Work and Standardize It

The father of lean production, Taiichi Ohno, stated, "In the Toyota production system, sequencing of work and work standardization are done first. 'Efficient patient workflow' means that we provide defined value to the patient in each step of a process while the patient flows along. Moving the patient from place to place is in itself not continuous workflow but work forced to flow. Accomplishing as many steps as possible with minimal movement and transport between process steps is most efficient and constitutes 'continuous and efficient patient work flow.' In this way, most problem areas can be eliminated or improved."[17] Once the work sequence has been improved and standardized, additional improvements can follow with the purchase of better equipment where justified. Purchasing new or better equipment is one way of improving work. "But, if equipment improvement comes first, work processes will never be improved." One will often find that even an old, well-maintained piece of equipment will deliver good service with a lean process that flows continuously. After sequencing and standardizing processes to achieve continuous flow, allow each department the opportunity to review the adequacy of its equipment and surrounding physical environment. If it's clear that an improved instrument or piece of equipment or other physical change will significantly improve productivity, cost, or quality, provide a method to accurately analyze, prioritize, and approve such purchases as needed or at least annually, such as during the budgeting process. Do an ROI analysis on each request. Inadequate or faulty instruments, devices and equipment, or other elements of the physical work environment can hamper other process improvement steps. Use the right instruments and equipment and make them easily accessible. All too often, important instruments and equipment are not readily available or in proper working condition. But above all, sequence and standardize work to achieve lean production. Thirty years ago at the beginning of my career in healthcare, I believed that computers, automation, and new information systems were the ultimate solution for improving healthcare. Today I know that the real solution is to relentlessly pursue continuous process improvement. Computers, automation, and other new purchases are secondary to first improving work processes.

In Appendix D, Jennifer Condel, anatomic pathology team leader at the University of Pittsburgh Medical Center Shadyside Hospital, and her colleagues present an excellent case study of TPS in healthcare: "Error-Free Pathology: Applying Lean Production Methods to Anatomic Pathology." They show how the hospital uses Toyota continuous flow methods with the goal of reducing pathology process time from 48 hours to 24 hours (from obtaining the specimen to reporting the results). Credit is also due to Stephen S. Raab, MD, David T. Sharbaugh, and Karen Wolk Feinstein, PhD, as detailed in Appendix D. A related article, "Small Improvements Yield Big Results in Shadyside Pathology Lab," appears in the August 2004 newsletter on the Pittsburgh Regional Healthcare Initiative (PRHI) Web site.[18]

28 Eliminate Bottlenecks to Improve Continuous Flow

Eliyahu M. Goldratt's 2004 book, *The Goal,* is an enjoyable classic that emphasizes the continual elimination of bottlenecks to improve process flow.[19]

He explains that performance is improved by first locating and eliminating the primary bottleneck, which is limiting the overall throughput of a process. This will cause a different primary bottleneck to become visible. The process of sequentially eliminating bottlenecks continues until the value stream is optimized.

Goldratt states that the key motivation of every business is to "make money in the present as well as in the future." A hospital CEO that I knew would often say, "No money, no mission," which basically agrees with Goldratt's thesis. Goldratt contends that only three key performance measures ultimately matter:

1. Increased throughput (T)

2. Decreased inventory (I)

3. Decreased operating expense (OE)

All three contribute to improving the three most important financial measures:

1. Net profit

2. Return on assets or investment

3. Cash flow

All three of the above measures must be positive to make money. Business performance is improving when all three measures increase simultaneously.

The above six key measures should therefore be included in any organization's scorecard to monitor its ultimate performance.

We have measurements like net profits, ROI, and cash flow to assess bottom-line performance. We can also monitor throughput, inventory, and operating expenses as well to guide our progress. Goldratt defines these key measures in a way that is different from conventional accounting.

Throughput—The rate at which the system generates money through sales.

Inventory—All the money the system invests in purchasing things the system intends to sell.

Operating expense—All the money the system spends in turning inventory into throughput.

Goldratt's theory of constraints (that is, elimination of bottlenecks) continually focuses on:

What to change?

What to change to?

How to cause the change?

via:

1. Identifying the system's bottlenecks.

2. Deciding how to exploit or eliminate the bottlenecks.

3. Subordinating everything else to the above decision. Make sure that everything marches to the tune of the bottlenecks to achieve maximum throughput. Underusing a bottleneck area will severely limit overall performance.

4. Elevating the system's bottlenecks. Act as if they are your most important concern.

5. If, in a previous step, a bottleneck has been eliminated, going back to step 1.

Basically, Goldratt strives to improve performance by continually identifying, examining, and removing a primary bottleneck. By doing so one can move performance toward the ultimate goal of perfection. Using Goldratt's prescription to improve performance is a logical follow-up to any lean implementation.

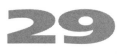 # Document All Important Processes in the Organization or Department

It's important to document standardized processes to ensure continued conformance. It's not necessary to adopt rigorous ISO 9001–type process documentation, but at least document all major processes and all significant improvements using your organization's policy/procedure format. Remember to include an up-to-date process flowchart. Document in detail how a standardized process is supposed to be executed every time to achieve the desired level of cost and quality. Without this documentation and a commitment to follow it consistently, the process will vary uncontrollably. Use the indicators on the scorecard discussed in step 11 to ensure that the new standard process is being effectively executed. In the following steps, we'll improve the "standard process" so that it functions with even higher quality and lower cost. After making improvements to a process, redocument it again in policy/procedure form. Use the scorecard to hold the gains and to confirm that you're doing so. Without a focused effort to hold the gains, a process will easily revert to prior variability, and hard-won improvements can be easily lost. Adopting ISO 9001 process documentation may be of interest to hold the gains, as there is a yearly audit to ensure that processes are actually being performed according to the documented standards.

An article on the ASQ Web site about the Physician's Clinic of Iowa (PCI)[20] in Cedar Rapids discusses its quality management system using the ISO 9001 format. Most healthcare organizations haven't fully embraced ISO, but this article gives some good insights into the development of an ISO quality management system for healthcare.

Certain departments can more easily benefit from an ISO quality system design, such as materials management and supply processing (SPD), surgery, radiology, lab, and pharmacy. These departments are more process and procedure oriented, and thus can more easily adopt an ISO quality system.

Focus on standardizing process steps and maintain those standards rather than reinventing the wheel each time to deal with situations. When staff change, ensure that the new staff are trained in the approved standards and documentation.

3O Implement and Maintain Continuous Improvement

The Japanese word for *continuous improvement* is kaizen. This is the small steps Toyota takes every day to continuously improve cost and quality. Kaizen involves continuous process improvement, elimination of waste, inventory reduction through just-in-time kanban techniques, total productive maintenance of all instruments and equipment to minimize breakdowns, policy deployment so that all employees understand the basic strategic plan, an active employee suggestion system, and ongoing team activities.

Organizations should define the methods and tools to be used for improvement activities and include them in the Quality and Cost Improvement manual and related training. Examples include:

- Identify each process owner. (This simple but critical step is often ignored. Identifying the process owner immediately assigns responsibility and accountability for improvement.)

- Educate the process owner about improvement methods.

- Define process boundaries.

- Establish functional and cross-functional improvement teams

- Train the teams in improvement methods.

- Use tools such as diagrams, statistical techniques, and check sheets to improve.

- Map key processes using flowcharts.

- Measure the effectiveness and efficiency of the system and continually improve.

It may be necessary to repeat steps 29 and 30 several times to achieve a final "standardized process." It may be necessary to first document a standardized process before being able to improve it using improvement techniques. After improvement, it will be necessary to re-document the newly improved standardized process. As continuous improvement occurs, these two steps of standardization and improvement may be repeated continuously until a desired standardized outcome is gradually achieved. Still continuous improvement does not stop there, since there is a relentless ongoing pursuit for perfection in the process.

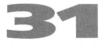 ## Consider Radical Improvement Where Appropriate

As you know, *kaizen* means continuous improvement. There is another Japanese word, *kaikaku,* which means radical improvement. Radical improvement may involve rearranging major processes in a single day with a doubling of productivity and a dramatic reduction in errors. This is similar to the concept of reengineering in the West. Often reengineering efforts stop at boundaries within the organization and consultants then collect their fees and leave. They fail to consider and improve the entire value stream for the patient or customer. They often treat employees as the enemy to be eliminated, which is contrary to our philosophy of respecting employees, helping develop them, and striving to retain them. Undertake reengineering efforts with great care and lots of open, honest communication. If well-performing staff are displaced, ensure that they have first preference for any open positions in the organization. Honor their contributions to the organization and maintain a long-term view of their continuing value to the organization.

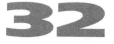 ## Videotape Each Step of Entire Work Processes

Videotaping is best, but at least photograph the steps from end to end to identify opportunities for improvement. A rapid improvement circle (RIC) then views the videotape repeatedly to identify alternatives for improvement, and applies the organization's quality and cost improvement methods. This videotaping may reenergize RIT or RICs if they are losing momentum. Typically, expensive consultants are hired to observe departmental processes and suggest ways to improve their cost and quality. It is possible to train a subgroup of a RIC or a subgroup of the hospital's internal quality and cost improvement department to do process observations and videotaping, make recommendations to the department head, and report progress. It's a good idea to include the department head or supervisor and RIC members as ad hoc members of this team. This departmental observation team may observe non-value-added activities, waste in all its forms, excess inventory, idle equipment and facilities, and underused employees. Videotaping is recommended to capture non-value-added activities and showcase improvements. New approaches are needed to stop skyrocketing healthcare costs and to simultaneously improve quality. It is better to implement an observation team from within than to hire one-time consultants who will eventually leave. Doing even a major cost reduction/quality improvement effort doesn't need to cost millions of dollars for consultants, and be a one-time effort, which will likely eventually evaporate. I am aware of several consultant-led quality and cost improvement engagements that cost several million dollars each and had transitory results. Improvement must be built into the organization. This can be done with a trained facilitator or two, one of whom may be the director of the existing internal quality and cost improvement department or a vice president, accompanied by the supporting structure described in Figure 3.2.

33 Use Flowcharts to Improve Core Processes

Core processes are the main customer value added processes of the business. Flowchart these important processes. Flowcharting software such as Microsoft Visio may assist, but hand-drawn flowcharts are adequate. A core process is defined as one of the primary processes the organization uses to achieve its mission or purpose. For example, the following are considered to be core processes for a hospital and need to be made as efficient as possible, as they represent the primary functions within the hospital. Each core process is labeled PVA if it is primarily patient (that is, customer) value added, or BVA if it is primarily business value added and not something a patient would normally choose to pay for.

Admission (BVA)

Emergency room treatment (PVA)

All patient scheduling processes (BVA), such as inpatient and outpatient

Outpatient treatment (PVA)

Ancillary testing, such as lab and x-ray (PVA)

Surgical treatment (PVA)

Medical treatment (PVA)

Nursing care process (PVA)

Therapy treatments (PVA)

Medication process (PVA)

Discharge (BVA)

Billing and administration (BVA)

It is important to remove all non-value-added steps and functions within these core processes as they represent waste. Ask yourself, "What would I as a patient be willing to actually pay for that step or activity or function?" Eliminate steps or functions that do not provide direct value to the patient or the business. Some process steps or functions may not be value added to the patient, but they may be business value added to the organization. They may be necessary for the organization to function appropriately. For example, the entire billing process and other administrative processes do not provide direct value to the patient, but they are necessary for the organization to survive. Still, business value-added processes need to be minimized and probably also contain many non-value-added steps that can be eliminated. Patient value-added processes must be made more efficient or even possibly increased if the patient desires.

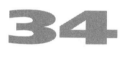 ## Use Spaghetti Diagrams to Trace the Path of a Patient, Employee, or Product

A spaghetti diagram is a diagram of a department or facility that shows the actual path taken by a patient or product as it moves through a process. A spaghetti diagram may also show all the steps and paths that workers follow to complete their jobs. All the starts and stops and the large distances traversed are sometimes very surprising. Strive for a final spaghetti diagram that minimizes starts and stops, waits, and distances. It should show a continuous, direct, and efficient flow.

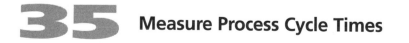 ## Measure Process Cycle Times

In addition to making flowcharts and spaghetti diagrams of important processes, measure cycle times within processes. Cycle time may be defined as "the total time it takes to complete a process step or a specific sequence of process steps." One can get a good sense of how well a process is working by just taking 5 to 10 cycle-time measurements of each step in the process as well as the entire process. This may not be statistically valid, but these observations will immediately give you a quick understanding of how well the process is working. If necessary, you can later do 30 to 100 cycle-time measurements of each step to get more precise understanding. Often, the initial quick and dirty 5 to 10 measurements will point out obvious opportunities.

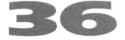 **Implement Quick Changeovers Within a Process**

A quick changeover allows a new process to resume with little delay, maximizing available resources. Examples are operating room, emergency room, and cath lab room turnover times between cases; procedure room turnovers in other ancillary departments like x-ray, nuclear medicine, and CT scan; lab draw cycle times between patients; and bed turnover time between patient departure and next patient arrival. Teach employees to distinguish between internal changeover times, which create a pause in the process, and external changeover times, which can be done in parallel with the process without halting it. To achieve best success, employees should form a quick changeover team led by an employee who has the best understanding of the changeover technology. They should set goals as a group to improve the changeover time by, for example, 50 percent. Picture a pit crew in a NASCAR race. It's amazing how fast the crew can return a racecar to the track. I'm sure it wasn't that way 50 years ago. Now, it may be a large crew in which everyone knows their duties; it may use technology like quick-fill fuel cans, lug wrenches that remove all the nuts from a wheel at the same time, and not just one such wrench but four working in parallel to change all four tires at once. Picture that type of pit crew commitment to turning over a cardiac surgery suite. A goal-setting method that encourages efficient changeovers is to post a sign that lists the names of quick-changeover team members, the leader's name, and the time it last took to perform the changeover, as well as the target time. Hang the sign for all to see.

When targets are achieved, the quick changeover team demonstrates for other staff how it's done. Present an award or achievement certificate to the team that makes the presentation.

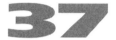 ## Complement Nursing Care Delivery Models with Lean

Healthcare providers use various nursing models to deliver patient care as defined in Table 3.3. Lean is complementary to all these models as it delivers true value to patients by eliminating various forms of waste.

Table 3.3 Models of nursing care delivery.

Nursing Care Delivery Models	Definition
Patient-Focused Care	A model popularized in the 1990s that used RNs as care managers and unlicensed assistive personnel (UAP) in expanded roles such as drawing blood, performing EKGs, and performing certain assessment activities
Primary or Total Nursing Care	A model that generally uses an all-RN staff to provide all direct care and allows the RN to care for the same patient throughout the patient's stay; UAPs are not used and unlicensed staff do not provide patient care
Team or Functional Nursing Care	A model using the RN as a team leader and LPNs/UAPs to perform activities such as bathing, feeding, and other duties common to nurse aides and orderlies; it can also divide the work by function such as "medication nurse" or "treatment nurse"
Magnet Hospital Environment/Shared Governance	Characterized as "good places for nurses to work" and includes a high degree of RN autonomy, MD–RN collaboration, and RN control of practice; it allows for shared decision making by RNs and managers

Source: Agency for Healthcare Research and Quality (http://www.ahrq.gov/clinic/ptsafety/chap39.htm). The Agency for Healthcare Research and Quality (AHRQ) is the lead federal agency charged with improving the quality, safety, efficiency, and effectiveness of healthcare for all Americans.

Some providers implement patient-focused care, which is further characterized by the following list of characteristics.

- Decentralized patient services located close to the patient's room to minimize patient transport

- Cross-trained nursing/tech/aide staff

- Consistent nursing-care teams per patient

- Standardized care and charting by exception

- Patient is center of everything

- Emphasis on patient satisfaction

It is easy to see the parallels between patient-focused care and lean, such as minimizing transport, using multiskilled staff, providing standardized care, and focusing on the patient/customer. Lean facilitates various nursing care models by delivering care more efficiently. Lean doesn't hamper good patient care. Rather, lean is simply a philosophy that facilitates effective patient care by making care delivery processes as efficient as possible. Lean helps caregivers deliver good patient care.

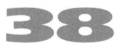 **Challenge and Work with Your Extended Network of Suppliers and Partners**

Help your suppliers and partners improve. Treat them as an extension of your own business. Map the flow from suppliers and partners all the way through to patient discharge. Together, improve process to achieve continuous flow between partners and you. Set challenging targets. Create continuous flows of small lots (hours rather than days) of supplies and materials from vendors. At a Toyota plant, there is less than an hour's worth of inventory next to each worker. This is made possible through the use of the continuous kanban supply system. Furthermore, suppliers deliver directly to the worker's station often sometimes hourly and certainly several times a day, with no inspection required. The inventory savings immediately fall to the bottom line. The lean assembler has no reserve stocks. A faulty shipment can be disastrous, but this almost never happens because the suppliers know what that can mean. And if a part is defective, the work team will immediately identify the cause to prevent a recurrence.

Toyota identifies a group of first-tier suppliers, in which Toyota retains a minority financial interest. The first-tier suppliers use second-tier suppliers, which are independent. Certify suppliers based on defects per million, so that no inspection is required on receiving. If their defect rates are excessive, transfer a portion of orders to other suppliers for a limited time until quality improves. Retain a cooperative relationship with all suppliers. Work with them as a team to continuously improve their processes and reduce their costs. Typically Toyota uses a third to an eighth as many suppliers as traditional U.S. automakers. Toyota's technique of single sourcing supplies is not just a matter of just selecting one supplier. It is rather the building of a long-term relationship based on a contract framework that encourages cooperation. Toyota works with the supplier to reduce the supply cost while maintaining the supplier's profit, or even allowing the supplier to receive an additional profit from a portion of any cost reduction achieved. The idea is for the lean assembler to work with the supplier so that the supplier can become a lean supplier. This is a fundamental shift away from the power-based negotiating present in U.S. industries.

Some healthcare suppliers may be clinical partners that refer patients to you. Ensure that the referral process is simple, quick, seamless, and as smooth as possible. To the extent possible, transfer all demographic and insurance information and medical records from the partner, so that you do not have to re-ask patient demographic and insurance questions. Expect that there will be no defects in the referral process and hold to this standard. Transfer information between information systems to help solve this problem, or consider new technology such as smart ID cards, which store patient information. Or just ask the partner to provide a printout to the patient containing all current demographic, insurance, and other information.

39 Automate Processes to Further Improve Quality and Cost

Improve processes first. Simplify value-added steps and eliminate all non-value-added steps. After processes have been manually improved and standardized, then it's time to automate. That is, first simplify and eliminate, then automate. Do a careful cost–benefit analysis of any proposal for automation. Be sure you are improving quality and/or reducing costs; otherwise, question why you are automating. Don't automate just for the sake of automation. First establish firm new goals for improved quality and cost. Beware of untested or "bleeding edge" technology, which may cause extreme process disruptions. Use only reliable, well-accepted technology, and be sure it is well tested and verified before proceeding. Conduct thorough pilot tests under similar conditions. You may find that automation just isn't worth it when you consider the cost of the additional equipment and of the labor and maintenance. Adopt automation carefully in sync with your specific goals to improve processes, improve quality, and reduce cost. After thorough analysis, quickly implement well-tested technologies that will improve flow in your processes.

40 Learn from Benchmark Nonhealthcare Organizations

Emulate Toyota, Ritz Carlton Hotels, Wal-Mart, McDonald's, and Disney. Don't just watch what they do. Make a focused effort to do what they do, and even improve upon it. Most of us are familiar with Wal-Mart. What can one learn from Wal-Mart? Some of the next points may not directly reduce cost but will improve quality as perceived by the customer and will increase market share without the need for expensive marketing and advertising. Kmart was near bankruptcy because of the customer-oriented practices Wal-Mart uses to increase quality and market share.

What can hospitals learn from Wal-Mart?

- Wal-Mart has a greeter who invariably says, "Welcome to Wal-Mart." When did you last hear "Welcome," or when did you at least feel welcome as you entered a hospital?

- If you ask where something is located at Wal-Mart, an associate courteously takes you there without hesitation. Does that regularly happen in your hospital?

- Wal-Mart has a no-hassle price-matching policy. If you can show any ad from a local store for the same item, Wal-Mart will match the price, no questions asked. Actually, the chain goes beyond simple price matching. It posts the ads from local competitors on a bulletin board near the store's main entrance. A customer need only look at all the ads and then ask for a price match. Has any healthcare provider ever done price matching like that, even though procedure costs vary greatly among providers? Have any providers ever posted competitors prices for easy comparison in a public area? I highly doubt it. I once asked a healthcare provider to quote a price for a procedure, and after about 20 minutes I was given a handwritten scrap of paper with a wide range of costs written on it that I found difficult to understand. I wasn't impressed. I wouldn't have accepted that from an automobile body, brake, or muffler shop, but I was forced to accept it from the healthcare provider. As a customer, I did not feel I was well served, and I would be delighted in the future if a healthcare provider were able to quickly provide accurate cost estimates for services.

- Wal-Mart has a no-hassle return policy if the customer is dissatisfied for any reason. I bought a jacket at Wal-Mart, and after a couple of months the zipper stopped working. I took it back and quickly and courteously received a new jacket, without any questions. Another time, I bought some cheese on sale at the Wal-Mart food store. When I got home, I noticed that it rang up on the register receipt at regular price. Since the store is only a couple blocks away from my home, I returned it later that afternoon. They didn't just refund the difference, but actually gave me the cheese for free as it was their own pricing error. If there were an error on a healthcare bill, would the provider just refund the difference or do something more to compensate for the patient's trouble in calling attention to the error? Also, if a healthcare procedure has some untoward outcome, like an infection, do healthcare providers promptly and courteously offer to refund the procedure cost or do corrective follow-up procedures for free?

- I have been impressed by Wal-Mart's return policies, and lately I am wondering if their return policy ever disagrees with a customer's desires. I have begun to feel like testing the limits of their great customer service to see if they will disappoint rather than delight me as a customer. Most recently I bought a sealed package of six bars of hand soap, and I found that I was allergic to it. Of course, I had had to open and use a bar to find that out. I returned the unopened five bars with the broken cellophane packaging around them and explained that I was allergic to it. I explained that one bar was missing, since that was the one I used. Well, what do you think? They accepted the five returned bars, and refunded me the full original price for the package of six. So, I remain impressed with Wal-Mart's customer service policies to this day, and must say I'm delighted.

- The outside signs at my Wal-Mart say "Always low prices" above the entrance. How many healthcare providers have a slogan like "Always low prices?" Many might say "Always rising prices at 3 to 6 times the rate of general inflation."

- Most Wal-Marts are open 24 hours a day and seven days a week. The sign above one entrance says "Always Food Center." That's called a "good access" strategy. The other supermarket a few blocks away, which closes at 10 P.M., had five cars in its parking lot at 9:30 P.M. while the Wal-Mart had about 50 cars in front of its food store and another 50 in front of its discount store. The competitor will be lucky to survive unless it quickly changes.

- Wal-Mart is clean and well organized with pleasant music playing in the background. It has a large, well-lighted parking lot. It combines a discount store, food store, pharmacy, photo center, auto service center, gas station, and snack bar, along with several boutique shops (eyeglasses, hair styling) at the main entrance. This is one-stop shopping. A customer can satisfy nearly all of his or her shopping needs with one stop without undue waiting. How often do patients have most of their needs filled with one stop? More commonly, patients may not be able to see a particular physician for weeks and then may be referred to another physician, for whom they must similarly wait for weeks to see, often at a different location. For example, patients in Boston wait on average more than a month to see medical specialists, the longest wait in a survey of 15 major cities. The shortest wait, of eight to 15 days, was in Washington, DC.[21] How many physicians and hospitals have "open access" appointment systems that can give a patient an appointment on the very day they call? How often do you hear or read about emergency rooms packed with patents waiting hours to be seen? In April 2002, the Associated Press reported that one in three hospitals was diverting ambulances due to overcrowding in their emergency rooms. These are examples of "poor access" strategies for healthcare services.

- If you get your car's oil changed at Wal-Mart, workers will also vacuum the interior and wash the windshield. This is an example of giving customers more than they expect. This strategy will often delight a customer and encourage their return. How often do patients receive services that delight them and encourage them to be return customers?

- As I finish the checkout at Wal-Mart, the cashier may say "Thank you, Robert" after observing my name on my credit or debit card. How often do hospital employees call patients by their names, or do they more often treat patients as numbers? Customer service training should be required for all new healthcare employees, and it should be periodically refreshed for existing employees. Ritz Carlton, for example, trains every new employee for days to "become ladies and gentlemen" before they even begin their job.

And what can hospitals learn from McDonald's? McDonald's has become an icon of American culture, almost like Coca-Cola. How did it become so successful? It all started over 50 years ago when Ray Kroc traveled to San Bernadino, CA, to learn why a small hamburger stand had ordered 10 of the milkshake mixing machines he was selling. They must be doing something special to need this big order.

What Ray Kroc saw in San Bernadino in 1955 was Richard and Maurice McDonald making hamburgers more efficiently than anyone else using their "Speedee Service System." Ray believed he could replicate this best practice in his home state of Illinois and other parts of the United States, and McDonald's was born. Retired coaches can remember taking a busload of basketball players to McDonalds in the 1960s and ordering 100 hamburgers and 50 or 60 orders of fries, and amazingly getting their order in about 10 minutes. And, the kids liked it.

Kroc insisted that his McDonald's restaurants look the same and that all staff follow the same procedures across the country to produce the same high-quality product at an affordable price. Now people going to McDonald's from Boston to Beijing know what they are going to get. They simply want reliable, predictable, high-quality and reasonably priced products and services—the same thing that hospital patients want.

Early on McDonald's listened to its customers. In the 1950s and '60s automobile ownership was rising fast and more mothers were working. McDonald's filled these customers' needs for easy access and speedy service and at the same time catered to public tastes. Is healthcare adequately responding today to its customer needs?

What have been the results of McDonalds' standardization, speed, reasonable cost, and meeting customer's needs with predictable service quality? The small chain that started in the 1950s now boasts more than 30,000 restaurants serving 50 million people a day. McDonald's is still a high-performing business example today with a 15 percent jump in profits in 2006 to $2.6 billion. It has adjusted to the times with healthier salad options and has launched a campaign to teach children about the benefits of healthy eating and exercise. Hospitals and other healthcare providers can similarly become successful by standardizing their business practices and streamlining their operations and by simply listening to the needs of their customers.

41 Learn from Other Benchmark Healthcare Organizations

Also learn from Baldrige Award finalists and winners. What is the Malcolm Baldrige National Quality Award?

The Baldrige Award is given by the President of the United States to businesses—manufacturing and service, small and large—and to education and healthcare organizations that apply and are judged to be outstanding in seven areas: leadership, strategic planning, customer and market focus, information and analysis, human resource focus, process management, and business results.

Between 1987 and 2006 there were 51 Baldrige Award recipients from over 9,500 applicants. The Baldrige Award for Healthcare was established in 1999. Over 50 Baldrige Healthcare applications have been submitted since its inception and there have been a total of six Baldrige awards in healthcare.[22] In 2002 the Franciscan Sisters of Mary Health Care (SSMHC) based in St. Louis, Missouri, received the first Baldrige award for healthcare. SSMHC is composed of 21 hospitals and three nursing homes located through out the Midwest. Any healthcare organization can learn from SSMHC, and for that matter it can use the same Baldrige criteria and application to improve, even if it doesn't apply for the Baldrige Award.[23]

In a 2007 press release on its Web site, SSMHC stated, "Since 1999, SSMHC has exceeded its charity care goal of contributing a minimum of 25 percent of its operating margin (before deductions) from the prior year. These contributions are used to provide care to people who cannot pay." This is an example for every hospital in America to emulate. Possibly Congress should consider a bill that would require each hospital to similarly contribute a certain percentage of its operating margin (that is, profit) or cash reserves to charity care in order to maintain its not-for-profit corporate status. This would help provide some relief to the growing numbers of uninsured.

Similarly, Baptist Health Care (BHC) of Pensacola, Florida, is recognized as one of the nation's truly outstanding healthcare organizations, for both staff and patients. BHC has ranked among the 15 best employers, according to *Fortune* magazine's annual "100 Best Companies to Work for in America" list. The companies are selected from a large national pool of candidate organizations and ranked based principally on how a random selection of employees responded to a survey that measures the quality of their workplace culture. Completing the patient–employee connection, Baptist Health Care has been in the top 1 percent in perceived patient satisfaction, from research conducted among hospitals nationwide. Today, Baptist Health Care has one of the lowest hospital annual staff turnover rates in the nation (just over 14 percent) and one of the highest levels of employee morale for any company in any industry.[25]

Notice, however, that achieving a current staff turnover rate in the low teens still means that about one in eight employees is leaving BHC annually. That implies large rehiring costs, which aren't patient value added. More improvement is needed. Imagine what levels of turnover less successful hospitals are experiencing. In addition, other awards and notable distinctions Baptist Health Care has earned include:

- The *USA Today* Quality Cup for extraordinary results in employee and patient satisfaction

- The highest hospital employee morale in the country, as reported by a nationally syndicated employee attitude study

- The National Leadership Award for Excellence in Patient Care from Voluntary Hospitals of America

- Finalist visits for the Malcolm Baldrige National Quality Program in 2000, 2001, and 2002

How does the Baldrige Award differ from ISO 9000?

The purpose, content, and focus of the Baldrige Award and ISO 9000 are very different. The Baldrige Award was created by Congress in 1987 to enhance U.S. competitiveness. The award program promotes quality awareness, recognizes quality achievements of U.S. organizations, and provides a vehicle for sharing successful strategies. The Baldrige Award criteria focus on results and continuous improvement. They provide a framework for designing, implementing, and assessing all business operations.

ISO 9000 is a series of five international standards published in 1987 by the International Organization for Standardization (ISO), which is based in Geneva, Switzerland. Companies can use the standards to help determine what is needed to maintain an efficient quality conformance system. For example, the standards describe the need for an effective quality system, for ensuring that measuring and testing equipment is calibrated regularly and for maintaining an adequate record-keeping system. ISO 9000 registration determines whether a company complies with its own quality system.

Overall, ISO 9000 registration covers less than 10 percent of the Baldrige Award criteria, since it provides little encouragement for continuous improvement. Organizations with advanced quality systems can still consider it especially for its yearly audit of standardized processes.

42 Learn from the Institute For Healthcare Improvement

In addition to the above steps, refer to the Institute for Healthcare Improvement (IHI) as a valuable source for cost reduction and quality improvement ideas [http://www.ihi.org]. IHI hosts free Internet e-mail groups on topics such as "Idealized Design of Clinical Office Practices," which can be invaluable in helping improve healthcare quality and cost. IHI's publications and collaboratives also tackle many of the problems within healthcare. IHI sponsors several initiatives, which focus on core problems. Some of these IHI initiatives may be independently pursued. However, pursuing IHI's individual initiatives does not take the place of building a permanent internal structure for continuous quality improvement and cost reduction as described in this book.

43 Hold on to the Gains You've Achieved

All too often, consultants or improvement projects become successful, but after a couple of years the gains evaporate. Consultants leave and gains slowly disappear. More than once, I have observed the gains from multi-million-dollar engagements dissipate within a few years. Or, improvement teams work hard to achieve meaningful gains, and then when they disband or change their focus, their gains slowly disappear. So a critical and often overlooked step is to put measures in place to hold your gains permanently. This may mean continuing to monitor the improvement via your finance or quality and cost improvement departments, or via a periodic scorecard that includes monitoring measures. Better yet, permanently build your improvements into the new process. It may mean documenting a new standard procedure and posting it at the job station. It may mean training each new employee in that standard procedure. It may mean a periodic review, audit, or training update to ensure that the standard procedure is being followed. Good documentation of newly improved methods and procedures using the organizations policy and procedure format is important to maintain any improvement. It is a good idea for employees to review process documentation at least annually and to discuss any deviations with the team leader (supervisor). The last thing you want is for gains to slowly evaporate or for a new team to come along a couple of years later, misunderstand the situation, and change the procedure back to a less effective one.

44 Reduce Administrative Overhead Costs

We talked earlier about increasing patient value-added care and simultaneously reducing administrative costs and other non-value-added costs within healthcare organizations. While performing each of the preceding 43 improvement steps, healthcare providers should be continuously increasing the percentage of dollars spent on direct patient value-added care as a portion of total expenses. It's fairly straightforward for any healthcare CFO to compute total salary dollars for hands-on value-added care givers. Total expenses are also easily obtained. Then it's a simple matter to just continually try to increase the percentage of direct-care dollars divided by total dollars spent. Doing so will increase true value-added services and decrease non-value-added services. It's also important to continuously confirm that the direct-care services being provided are truly value added for the patient and contain little or no waste.

45 Avoid Insurance Company Overhead Costs

We know that the United States spends almost $2 trillion annually on healthcare. Of this, possibly 20 percent is wasted on insurance company profits and their excess overhead costs. That may amount to $400 million that can be redirected to true patient value-added services. The profits and excesses of health insurance companies are dollars that are being directed away from real patient care. This can be corrected by taking whatever steps are necessary to avoid excessive insurance company overhead, such as the following:

1. Self-insuring companies that are large enough.

2. Moving more of the population under Medicare.

3. Implementing universal health coverage for children, or at least within some states.

4. Expanding state-sponsored insurance plans that demonstrate success, such as Massachusetts or Maine.

5. Moving more of the population under the same insurance plan that government workers and legislators enjoy.

6. Moving toward a single-payer system that eliminates excessive overhead and paperwork.

7. Implementing universal health coverage for all or most of the U.S. population, as all other developed countries enjoy.

8. Implementing a hybrid health insurance plan similar to France's, which guarantees a basic level of care to the entire population and yet allows citizens to purchase private plans to improve their health coverage. This may be the best of both worlds. Canada also seems to be drifting slightly in this direction. Maybe the United States should, too.

Doing the above could potentially reduce our $2 trillion U.S. national health expenditures by 15 percent to 20 percent, which is enough to cover all the uninsured in the United States. Of the remaining 1.6 trillion dollars of annual U.S. health expenditures, another 30 percent to 40 percent or $.6 trillion can be saved by eliminating all remaining waste within U.S. healthcare processes. Former U.S. Treasury Secretary Paul O'Neill has stated that approximately 50 percent of $2 trillion spent annually on healthcare can be eliminated by implementing principles used by lean manufacturing plants such as Toyota. These actions would leave the United States with a less expensive healthcare system focused on providing true value added services to all.

46 Take a Total Systems View of Healthcare for Lean Improvement

A closing improvement step is to take a total systems view of all opportunities to improve healthcare cost and quality and apply lean principles to each. Opportunities for reducing cost and improving quality are listed below in approximate decreasing order of magnitude. This is a Pareto-type approach, which identifies the greatest opportunities for improvement and then addresses each in approximate order of potential impact. Focus initially on the greatest opportunity, which is eliminating all forms of waste, and work through the list, applying lean to each opportunity. Use community, regional, state, and national scorecards to monitor improvement progress. Note that we can start eliminating waste in healthcare now without any political action or outside approval. Following is a list of opportunities for improvement:

1. Waste is rife within the healthcare delivery system. Experts like Dr. Donald Berwick estimate that 40 percent of healthcare processes represent waste to be removed. Hospital-related processes are the largest component, at about 32 percent of total healthcare costs.[†]

2. Insurance company overhead is 20 percent to 30 percent of all healthcare dollars spent and represents the second largest component to improve.

---

†Note—the percentages that follow total 100% when added to the hospital percentage of 32%

3. Physician practices represent 22 percent of total healthcare expenses and are candidates for improvement. It is amazing to note that insurance company overhead rivals the cost of all physician care.

4. Prescription drugs represent 9 percent of total healthcare expenses.

5. Nursing home services represent 7 percent of total healthcare expenses.

6. Medicare/Medicaid programs add 3 percent overhead costs and can be made more cost and quality efficient.

7. All other suppliers and contributors to healthcare cost and quality, such as medical supplies, equipment, and maintenance, can benefit from lean improvements.

8. Improve information flow to further enable lean. Not sharing information among healthcare providers often results in duplicate tests and procedures and delayed care. Computer automation is an enabler. Conversely, excessive computer automation can be a barrier to lean processes. Analyze carefully. Simplify first, and later automate.

9. State-sponsored healthcare programs can also be more lean and efficient, including children's healthcare programs. Target to minimize administrative costs.

10. Medical education and access to appropriate care remain overarching opportunities for lean improvement.

11. As all the above lean opportunities are pursued, let's not forget to lower individual healthcare costs by dietary, lifestyle, and exercise changes. Poor choices may indeed be root causes for much of our excess costs. Some companies promote exercise, diet, and lifestyle improvements by helping fund health club memberships, by reducing successful employees' health insurance rates, or by providing other incentives. One of the best ways to reduce healthcare is to ask "why it is needed" five times to get at the true root cause and to eliminate the need by lifestyle changes when possible.

4

A Capsule Summary of a Lean Toyota-like Production System for Healthcare

What follows is a capsule summary of the characteristics of a lean Toyota-like production system (TPS) that we are trying to implement in healthcare. At the core of a lean TPS is respect for employees. It means encouraging employees to make improvements to their jobs and the organization and respecting everyone's opinions. It means taking a long-term view of their employment and doing everything in your power to retain good employees and if necessary deploy them elsewhere in the organization where they can continue to provide continued good value.

Beyond the core of "respect for employees" are the following key activities within lean TPS:

1. Embed a permanent structure for cost and quality improvement in the organization (see Figure 3.2). This is a most important and critical action. This structure will automatically and relentlessly function every day to continuously improve healthcare quality and cost. It begins with a constant, clear, and visible commitment from every member of the organization's leadership, starting with the CEO, to continuously improve quality and reduce costs. It utilizes small Toyota-style work teams of three to eight cross-trained employees with a team leader who facilitates and shares in their tasks. It uses a group leader (that is, manager or supervisor) over multiple teams, totaling

approximately *60 employees. It includes board-sponsored strategic goals and teams to achieve those strategic cost and quality goals in a timely manner. It includes a rapid improvement steering team (RIT) of all managers and supervisors to jump-start lean. They learn to be lean leaders and to cultivate lean among their employees. Rapid improvement quality circles (RICs) of volunteer employees meet periodically on company time to continually improve quality and cost. Ask each employee on a RIC to submit one to four suggestions for cost and quality improvement per month and reward them appropriately. Later ask every employee in the organization to submit one or two suggestions per month. RICs evaluate the suggestions concerning their areas of responsibility. They also foster specific kaizen improvement efforts that may last from a day to a month.

2. Establish an improvement plan with goals accomplished by specific people and dates. Include in that plan your benchmark targets. Support this plan with empathetic "change management" for affected employees.

3. Establish an award/recognition/reward/gain-sharing program to encourage all to participate in cost and quality improvement. The hospital board approves this program to support its strategic objectives. Thank people publicly and repeatedly for their good contributions. Express sincere appreciation.

4. Create a simple, easy-to-understand quality and cost improvement manual to educate every employee. Publish an annual quality report to be reviewed alongside the annual financial report.

5. Educate all employees about the organization's strategic plan, and be sure they document their personal goals and understand how they contribute to the strategic plan.

---

*Note that a team leader does annual employee evaluations for their 8 team members, so the group leader (manager) only has to do annual evaluations for their 8 team leaders—no one is faced with doing 60 employee evaluations annually.

6. Create continuous flow. This means that the patient will easily move through the system with no waits and delays. The patient will immediately pull value-added activities to themselves as they move through the system of care and treatment. Use tools like direct observation teams, videotaping, flowcharts, value stream maps, and spaghetti diagrams to achieve continuous flow. Measure and continuously improve cycle times of process steps. Identify bottlenecks and continually remove them.

7. Sequence work and standardize it. This means having a standard best-practice way of doing each process step, clearly documenting it, and having that documentation clearly visible at the location where the process step is performed. Train each employee to perform the process steps in the standardized fashion.

8. Implement quick changeovers of rooms, staff, and equipment within process steps to minimize downtime.

9. Create "quality in station." This means that each worker at a process step creates no errors or defects, and the same worker who is performing a process step also does inspections to ensure high quality. Very little and preferably no follow-up inspection is needed, and no defects are passed to the next step.

10. Create a system for any employee to immediately stop/fix a defective process by immediately informing the team leader (supervisor) and/or group leader (manager) by personal contact, phone, page, or other immediate signal. Correct the process immediately so that the defect will not occur again.

11. Constantly eliminate waste in all its forms. This means eliminating all non-value-added steps that an uninsured patient would not choose to pay for. Define true value from the point of view of the patient (customer).

12. Reduce inventory and supplies to minimum levels that are still safe. This means providing inventory and supplies in small quantities when and where they are needed. Recall

that two hours of inventory is typical in Toyota's production system. Certainly organizations should avoid having weeks or months of inventory. Kanban signals provide inventory and supplies to processes at the rate that those processes use them up.

13. Create a visual workplace. This means that a casual observer can see all the work being done. This entails a reduction in private office space so the value-added activities of each employee are visible. It also means having equipment, instruments, inventory, and supplies well organized, visible, and easily accessible to employees.

14. Challenge and work with your extended network of suppliers and partners. Help them improve with you.

15. Hold your gains. Build your improvements into a well-documented standard process. Use a simple periodic scorecard to ensure that your hard-earned improvements do not evaporate. Enlist your finance department and your cost and quality improvement department to sustain your improvements and ensure that they are built to last.

16. After focusing on internal process improvements and achieving them, consider additional automation to further improve quality and cost. First simplify, then improve processes, and afterward automate. Be sure to do a cost–benefit analysis on every new capital purchase.

17. Reduce administrative overhead within the healthcare organization and avoid excess overhead from insurance companies. Eliminate all sources of waste to maximize value-added services for patient care. Take a total systems view of all the contributors to healthcare cost and quality and apply lean principles to each of them.

5

A Short To-Do List to Nationally Improve U.S. Healthcare Cost and Quality

1. Begin now to implement the "46 Steps to Improve Healthcare Quality and Cost" that are presented here. Permanently build the structure for cost and quality improvement into your organization, as shown in Figure 3.2, and maintain it. Eliminate all forms of waste (muda) and non-value-added activities. Focus on doing only value-added steps that an uninsured patient would actually choose to pay for. Continuously and relentlessly pursue quality and cost improvement. Certain hospitals in the United States are much more efficient than others. Copy known best practices within the United States and worldwide (for example, Baldrige winners and other healthcare and non-healthcare benchmark performers).

2. Write your senators and representative and lobby for national "ideally designed" hospital and clinic demonstration sites. Our government should support at least one U.S. hospital system and clinic to become a "demonstration site" for what can be achieved in highest quality and lowest cost. This project might be sponsored by IHI and supported by other quality and lean production experts. Encourage the use of industrial engineers and process improvement engineers to help improve healthcare, just as they helped Toyota and other companies improve. Many like me would welcome the opportunity to participate. Create clear incentives to reduce cost and improve quality. Our government could form a national team to replicate the results of the demonstration site to other interested healthcare

providers throughout the United States. Alternatively, the American Hospital Association (AHA) or the Voluntary Hospital Association (VHA) could help sponsor or replicate a demonstration site. If this demonstration site is not likely to be sponsored at a national level, then lobby for your state government or state hospital association to improve healthcare for your state. If that's unlikely, then strive for your own healthcare system to achieve demonstrate-site status so that others may see and emulate what you and your team have achieved. Then all other healthcare providers would be able to achieve similar world-class levels of quality and low cost. If voluntary improvement is not forthcoming, state or national legislation to improve cost and quality may be necessary. Then there will be hope for the United States to achieve better than its current World Health rank of 37th in "health system performance," without spending almost twice per capita on healthcare as any other nation in the world.

3. Stay tuned to changes and direction of national healthcare policy. Support new initiatives to reduce the 46 million uninsured in the United States and clamor for reduced healthcare costs. Lobby to reduce non-value-added activities, administrative costs, defects, medical errors, and pharmaceutical costs. Primarily reducing all waste and secondarily avoiding high insurance company overhead provide the greatest cost savings opportunities. Support a system that improves access to the underserved. Support importation or mass negotiation for cheaper pharmaceutical drugs. As we are the only developed country in the world without national health insurance, carefully evaluate and consider that option, or at least consider a single-payer system like Maine or Massachusetts.

4. Write your senators and representatives and lobby for completion of a certificate of need (CON) before any major new healthcare capital expenditure. This will help reduce growing duplication of equipment, services, and construction. If a national CON process is not likely, at least lobby to implement a CON process within your state. Too often city or county officials face decisions about choosing construction projects between volatile healthcare competitors, which is a decision they should not have to face.

5. Ask for a healthcare scorecard for your community. The National Committee for Quality Assurance (NCQA) and the United Way appear to support making these scorecards available online.[1]

Work with NCQA, the United Way, or similar organizations to use and expand these scorecards to improve the status of healthcare in your community and region. Ask the board members of your local healthcare providers what they are doing by when to improve community health status indicators.

6. It's time for all U.S. healthcare providers to rapidly reduce cost and improve quality by implementing the lean production steps described in this book. Implementing lean production is an effective strategy for achieving value and quality leadership in healthcare. High-quality healthcare may then be more affordable for all.

Appendix A
Automaker Benchmarks

Comparing the best

Key productivity and other operating measures for leading assembly plants run by major automakers in the United States:

Automaker	Toyota	Honda	Nissan	GM	Ford	Chrysler
Plant location	Georgetown, Ky.	East Liberty, Ohio	Smyrna, Tenn.	Lansing Grand River, Mich.	Kansas City, Ka.	Toledo, Ohio
Products	Toyota Camry, Avalon, Sienna, Camry Solara convertible	Honda Civic, Element	Nissan Altima, Frontier, Xterra	Cadillac CTS sedan	Ford Escape, Mazda Tribute, Ford F-150 pickup	Jeep Liberty
2002 assembly employment	4,849	2,327	3,632	749	5,563	2,307
2002 output (in units)	490,618	222,742	409,806	47,072	518,137	225,703
Labor hours per vehicle	22.81 ('01) 20.85 ('02)	19.20 ('01) 21.43 ('02)	17.92 ('01) 16.83 ('02)	Plant not in operation ('01) 32.35 ('02)	Escape/Tribute line 22.54 ('01) 22.1 ('02); F-150/Blackwood line 24.88 ('01) 24 ('02)	26.11 ('01) 24.02 ('02)
Capacity utilization rate* *Rate over 100 percent indicates plant ran on overtime	94% ('01) 104% ('02)	97% ('01) 91% ('02)	85% ('01) 94% ('02)	Plant not in operation ('01) 57% ('02)	Escape/Tribute line 125% ('01) 124% ('02); F-150/Blackwood line 112% ('01) 123% ('02)	102% ('01) 122% ('02)
Initial quality Problems per 100 cars in first 90 days of ownership	110 (Camry/Solara) 145 (Avalon) 123 (Sienna)	121 (Civic) 134 (Element)	130 (Altima) 151 (Frontier) 174 (Xterra)	88 (CTS)	141 (Escape) 151 (Tribute) 117 (F-150)	145 (Jeep Liberty)
Intangibles	• Has consistently built the popular Toyota Camry, among the most profitable, high-quality vehicles in Toyota lineup. • Has low absenteeism. • Has managed to overcome loss of key managers to rivals in recent years. • First Toyota plant in North America equipped with new welding system, the Global Body Line. • Consistently among most-utilized plants in U.S.	• Relied on overtime to prepare for Element launch, cope with West Coast strike by dock workers, which caused two down days. • Still consistently among most-utilized plants in U.S. • Has low absenteeism.	• Relies on high degree of automation in body shop, where steel skeleton is welded and assembled. • Also relies heavily on delivery of parts in sequence as needed, which eliminates excessive stockpiles. • Low absenteeism.	• Latest model of GM's manufacturing blueprint. • New plant and all-new product in 2002. • Very successful launch, met launch and quality targets. • One-shift operation. • Now builds Cadillac SRX SUV and preparing to build next generation STS sedan. • Cooperative, dedicated work force and labor union.	• Lincoln Blackwood output shelved in August 2002. • Ford's most productive pickup truck plant, despite higher, more complicated mix of content featured on trucks assembled in Kansas City. • One of Ford's most-utilized factories. Loyal, dedicated, focused, and cooperative workforce and labor union.	• Newest Chrysler plant and already among automaker's most-flexible plants, with ability to build diesel and right-hand drive versions of Liberty. • Slated for new expansion that will provide flexibility to build additional light truck products for Jeep.

*Rate over 100 percent indicates plant ran on overtime. Note: Mercedes-Benz and BMW do not participate in Harbour and Associates study; Civic and Camry quality scores include models assembled at other plants; plants selected through a variety of expert sources, automakers. Toyota's Georgetown plan stopped building the Sienna minivan in December 2002. *Sources:* Harbour and Associates, J.D. Power and Associates.
Source: Reproduced with permission of *The Detroit News.*

Appendix B

Children's Hospital and Regional Medical Center Emergency Department Patient Flow—Rapid Process Improvement (RPI)

Application of Toyota Production System Principles of Continuous Flow and Pull

Credits to: George A. Woodward, MD, MBA, Larry Godt, Michele Girard, Kelly Fisher, Shaughna Feeley, Margaret Dunphy, Barb Bouché

PROBLEM STATEMENT

In early 2004, the Emergency Department (ED) at Children's Hospital and Regional Medical Center in Seattle, Washington, began a continuous performance improvement process in order to address the following issues:

- An inefficient and noncentralized model of care

- An increase in the ED overall patient Length of Stay (see Figure B.1)

- An increase in problem scores from the Family Experience Survey

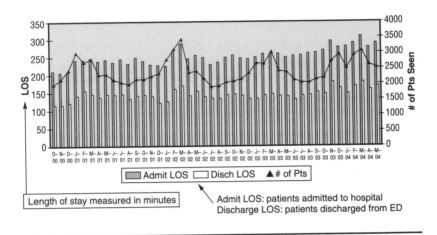

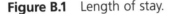

Figure B.1   Length of stay.

- Communication issues with the Referring Provider community

- Issues with continuum of care between community providers and hospital managment

Specifically, the ED wanted to:

- Improve the quality of care for patients based on data from the Family Experience Survey

- Improve efficiency of care, while decreasing waste in the system

- Improve communications with our Referring Community Physicians

- Ensure medical information capture between community, ED, and hospital providers

- Decrease ED patient length of stay

In addition, the ED would be moving into a new facility in 2007, and there was a desire to make corresponding improvements for the new facility.

INTERVENTION

A four-day RPI workshop was held in July 2004 in which the ED designed a new model of care. The ED implemented the work cell model in early December 2004 to provide more focused care, including the following elements:

1. Work cells called "pods (or zones)" were created. See Figure B.2.

   - Complex, Medium, and Fast pods/zones were created, based on historical and anticipated patient complexity and available supervision qualifications. Each pod/zone was staffed with an appropriate ratio of nurses, MDs, and Care Coordinators to treat the measured (and projected) volume of patients and required interventions in these pods. Staff such as Social Workers and Child Life Specialists were appropriately scheduled and located so as to provide a shared resource to all "pods."

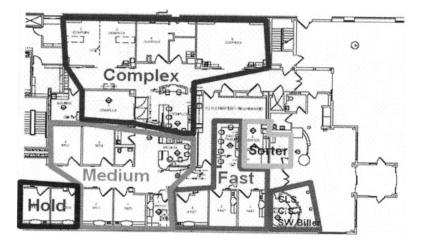

Figure B.2 New emergency department "pod design."

- A "pull" system was implemented that allowed for a better balance of patient demand to resource capability. As patients arrive in the ED, a provider completes a minimal intake to sort the patients based on acuity and assign them to a pod. ED related services and supplies are rapidly pulled to the ED patient based on their healthcare needs and associated orders.

- The design and location of the Fast, Medium, and Complex pods enable improved flow through the ED for patients and families. Teams of providers comprising the appropriate mix of disciplines work in assigned pods to facilitate the needed care for patients assigned to the pods.

2. Communications changes.

- A communication center was constructed and a Communication Specialist role was established to coordinate all incoming referrals, ED Team and in-hospital medical communications regarding expected or current patients, communication with and to Primary Care Providers (PCPs) regarding patient disposition and follow-up, as well as a notification system for when patients do not arrive as expected. This position is staffed 24/7 by an RN with additional communications training.

- An automated phone system was created to allow callers to choose the option that best fits their needs, including an option for the new communication center that coordinates all incoming communications from PCPs and medical transport teams en route to the ED.

3. Created a new patient chart for the ED. This "Uni-Form" combines both nurse and physician charting areas and replaces the multiple charting forms for patients.

During the first three months of implementation, the ED collected data to measure improvement in several key areas. This included measuring patient and staff satisfaction as well as ED length of stay. See Figures B.3 and B.4.

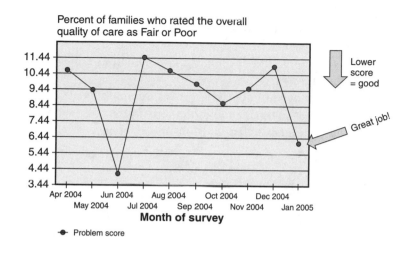

Figure B.3 Percent of families who rated the overall quality of care as fair or poor.

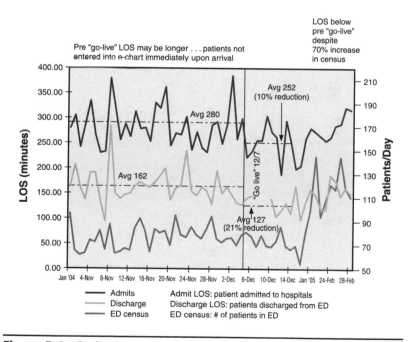

Figure B.4 Reduction in ED length of stay.

FOLLOW-UP ACTIONS

Upcoming actions include developing/implementing reliable methods as described below.

The ED team began Focused Events three months after implementation aimed at setting reliable methods in the following areas, which were identified as potential high-impact areas:

- Work balance among clinical and nonclinical staff

- Nursing role responsibilities

- Tasks assigned to Intake and Triage RNs

- Paperwork flow

- Lobby management

- Environmental Services support

- 5S projects

- Internal ED admission process

- Weekly Audits

- Communications

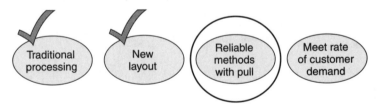

Appendix C

5S Catches on at the VA Pittsburgh Health System

(Sort, Set in order, Shine, Standardize, Sustain)

Credits to: VA Pittsburgh Healthcare System
Ellesha McCray, RN, Team Leader
Michael Moreland, CEO
Naida Grunden, Communications Director
Pittsburgh Regional Healthcare Initiative

Every business would like to improve productivity, reduce defects, meet deadlines, and provide everyone with a safer place to work. Yet in a complex hospital, making these kinds of major improvements might seem next to impossible.

At the 4 West Learning Unit at the VA Pittsburgh Healthcare System, staff discovered a relatively simple, rapid, low-cost, low-tech way of making these improvements. It's called 5S.

A LITTLE HISTORY

Before World War II, many American businesses had codified the idea that a clean workplace is a productive workplace. In America, by and large the idea remained in manuals, without being translated to the workplace. As Americans helped the Japanese reconstruct their industries after the war, they brought their ideas, and found the Japanese to be ready students. Before long, the Western idea of the orderly and productive workplace became tied to the Eastern idea of deep respect for the worker's well-being and morale. Out of this blend of philosophies came a technique for creating the orderly workplace, a technique directed not by a distant manager, but by the esteemed worker.

WHAT ARE THE FIVE S's?

The name, "5S," refers to a sequence of steps that translate approximately as follows:

Sort. Remove all items from the workplace that are not needed for current operations. A crowded workplace is hard to work in and costly to maintain.

Set in order. Arrange needed items so that they are easy to use. Label them so that they're easy to find, clean, and put away. This degree of order improves communication and reduces the frustration of wasted time and motion.

Shine. Clean the floors, walls, and equipment. When things are kept in top condition, when someone needs to use something, it is always ready. In a hospital environment, cleanliness is extremely important to staff member and patient alike.

Standardize. By integrating the first three steps into everyday work, "backsliding" is eliminated.

Sustain. If the rewards for keeping order outweigh the rewards for going back to the old way of doing things, people will make orderliness a habit.

PRACTICING 5S AT THE VA

About a year ago, the workers on 4 West, the inpatient surgical unit, took a long look at their equipment storage room. It looked like a typical storage room in any American hospital—a mix of often- and seldom-used equipment, stored in no particular order. It took time to find equipment, and it was difficult to walk around in the room. Items relying on recharged batteries were not always plugged in.

It wasn't clear where or in what condition things were supposed to be stored.

Following a deliberate process over a few weeks, staff members on 4 West were able to reduce the inventory in the room, while still maintaining access to what they needed when they needed it. About $20,000 worth of seldom used equipment was freed up for use in other areas of the hospital.

Signs clearly denote where each piece of equipment is to be stored, how it is to be cleaned, whether it is to be plugged in, and so on. The visual cues leave no doubt about the expectations.

Since the 5S, the room and equipment have been maintained in sparkling clean condition with little problem. Since cleaning is built into the work itself, backsliding is minimal.

So well has the equipment storage room worked that staffers on other units are now learning 5S. In short order, units on the fifth and sixth floors are organizing their storage rooms according to the principles.

"It's not just a matter of cleaning out your closet," says Peter Perreiah, PRHI's team leader at the VA. "It's about honoring the worker with a clean, safe environment, and honoring patients with equipment that's always clean and ready."

5S CATCHES ON

When she saw the equipment storage room on 4 West, Shedale Pinnix-Tindall, Nurse Manager on 6 West, thought it could work in her unit as well. Nobody asked her to do it. But she and Marianne Allen, 6 West Charge Nurse, asked for help and soon got started.

"Who could be against this? Having the storage areas orderly like this really saves time and frustration. It's better for patients," says Shedale, "and it's not hard to keep it this way."

Says Environmental Aide, John R. Finkley, "Since we did the 5S on 4 West, we can get what we need easily and quickly for every patient. There's no guessing. You just open the door and go right to the item. I find that I spend less time cleaning that room, so there's more time to clean every piece of equipment thoroughly. It's all part of the routine now."

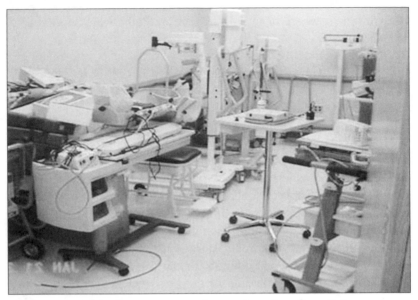

Figure C.1 Typical storage room in any American hospital.

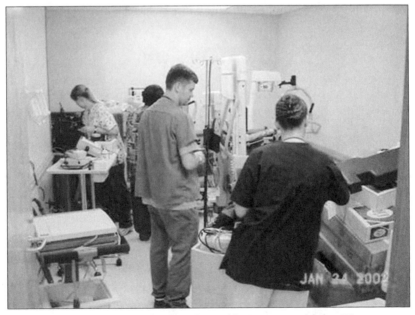

Figure C.2 Crew at VA Pittsburgh Health System amid the 5S process.

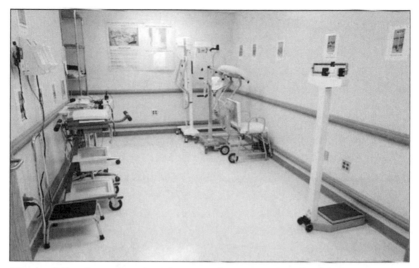

Figure C.3 Completed project. Wall posters visually delineate what goes where, how to clean and store.

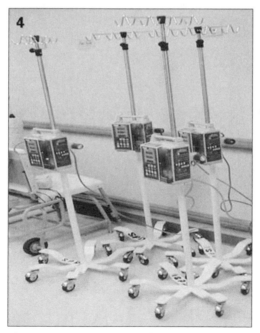

Figure C.4 Adequate electrical outlets mean equipment is always charged.

Appendix D

Error-Free Pathology: Applying Lean Production Methods to Anatomic Pathology

Jennifer L. Condel, BS, SCT(ASCP)MT,[a,*] David T. Sharbaugh, CPA,[b] Stephen S. Raab, MD[a]

[a]Department of Pathology, University of Pittsburgh Medical Center, Shadyside Hospital, Cancer Pavilion, 3rd Floor, 5150 Centre Avenue, Pittsburgh, PA 15232, USA
[b]University of Pittsburgh Medical Center, Presbyterian Shadyside Hospital, 5230 Centre Avenue, Pittsburgh, PA 15232, USA

By definition, "lean" refers to thin or sparse. In business, this word may have a negative connotation. The idea of "trimming the fat" or streamlining usually evokes the elimination of jobs. Employees therefore do not favor such techniques. At Toyota Motor Company, however, employees embrace "lean" as a work philosophy. This work ethic has developed through trial and error and evolved into the successful business practice known as the Toyota Production System (TPS). Lean methods, which include Six Sigma, strive to eliminate waste from a system. How this aim is accomplished varies among different methods, but one of the ultimate goals is a system that generates zero defects or errors.

This work was supported by the Jewish Healthcare Foundation, the Agency for Healthcare Research and Quality, and the University of Pittsburgh School of Medicine.

* Corresponding author.
E-mail address: condeljl@upmc.edu (J. L. Condel).

doi:10.1016/j.cll.2004.07.001   labmed.theclinics.com

Is error-free pathology possible? The authors think it is. If we do not challenge the current system and strive toward zero errors by experimentation, how will we know what is possible? This article is intended to share the authors' experiences in applying a lean production method to their anatomic pathology department, not only to reduce pathology errors to zero but to change a "blame culture" to one in which frontline staff members become effective problem solvers and the source of system improvements.

THE EVOLUTION OF LEAN

The phenomenon of lean business practice has drawn considerable attention over the last decade as a result of changing economics and customer demand. These same issues were the roots of the development of lean production after World War II, when Henry Ford's revolutionary manufacturing process of automobile mass production was practiced. The evolution of "lean" thinking may be traced through several generations of the Toyoda family. "They were innovators, they were pragmatic idealists, they learned by doing, and they always believed in the mission of contributing to society. They were relentless in achieving their goals . . . and they were leaders who led by example."[1]

An early example of lean thinking in the Toyoda family can be seen in the late 1800s, in the case of a carpenter and inventor named Sakichi Toyoda who designed wooden looms for weaving. Because the original design was labor-intensive, he strove to improve the looms for the women who used them. By 1926, Sakichi Toyoda had started the Toyoda Automatic Loom Works and successfully automated the loom using a steam engine. He is also credited with designing a mechanism by which the loom would automatically stop if a thread broke, thereby highlighting a problem. This practice of building quality into work, referred to as jidoka, enabled workers to perform value-added work and saved them from wasting time by watching machines work. From the root of this invention, jidoka became one of the two pillars of the lean production system known as TPS.[1]

In the early 1900s, an American named Henry Ford who was also interested in eliminating non-valued-added work created the cost-efficient process known as mass production for one style of automobile, the Model T. By incorporating people, materials, and machines in a continuous workflow design, Ford created cost-efficiency through simplicity: he synchronized the repetitive nature of tasks at each workstation, where only the materials needed were consumed.[2]

The Toyoda family advanced into the automotive industry when Sakichi Toyoda challenged his son Kiichiro to build an automobile business. Kiichiro Toyoda, a mechanical engineer, eventually built the Toyota Automotive Company and developed the idea of a "just-in-time" approach to work. This second pillar of TPS actually arose from Kiichiro Toyoda's trip to the United States, where he studied Ford's River Rouge automobile plant in Michigan and observed the replenishment system practiced in American supermarkets. The kanban replenishment system used in TPS is modeled after this process of "replacing products on the shelves just in time as the customers purchased them."[1] Kiichiro Toyoda's success was overshadowed after World War II; in 1948, he was faced with trying to prevent the company from going into bankruptcy as a result of overwhelming inflation. Toyoda's philosophy was not to fire employees under these circumstances. But his cost-cutting measures were inadequate, and he resigned as president, taking full responsibility for what he believed was his failure. Amazingly, other employees followed his lead and left voluntarily for the betterment of the company.

Kiichiro Toyoda continued to support the automobile industry by giving his cousin Eiji Toyoda, also a mechanical engineer, the task of establishing a "car hotel" (large parking garage) for a research laboratory. Toyota and other firms owned the "car hotel" for the purpose of supporting the small group of individuals who could still afford cars.[1] Eiji Toyoda researched the needs and supplies of the Toyota plant and ultimately became the president and chairman of Toyota.

MANUFACTURING COMPANY

Returning from a visit to Ford's Michigan plant in 1950, Eiji Toyoda gave Taiichi Ohno, a plant manager at that time, the task of "catching up with Ford's productivity."[1] Taiichi Ohno, Eiji Toyoda, and his managers spent 12 weeks studying the American plants. They observed what they believed were many system flaws and sources of waste, including disorganization and overhead as a result of excess inventory and large equipment needs. Taiichi Ohno was, however, impressed with Henry Ford's design of a continuous workflow assembly line that incorporated work standardization processes. Toyota's resources, unlike Ford's, were limited, and Taiichi Ohno knew Toyota needed to be able to produce small quantities of a variety of quality cars at the lowest cost in the shortest amount of time.

After World War II, customer demands changed and focused on variety. The American Big Three (Chrysler, General Motors, and Ford) responded to this change in demand by dismantling their original continuous flow design and switching to a process in which each portion of the assembly line functioned as an independent continuous flow entity. Taiichi Ohno viewed this form of mass production as introducing waste into the system. The process became more complex, requiring additional resources, and therefore was not an efficient way to meet the varied customer demands and maintain low production costs. Adopting Henry Ford's original workflow design, "a design that promoted efficiency by allowing work to flow continuously from beginning to end and by having it consume at every point only the resources needed to advance one unit of output one step further toward completion,"[3] Taiichi Ohno began to apply his learning to the shop floor where the work was done. The goal was to reduce waste or non–value-added work in the system, thus increasing employee satisfaction, quality, and productivity and maintaining low production costs. Through years of trial and error, working with the frontline staff, Taiichi Ohno and his team pioneered the lean production business practice known as TPS, which incorporated the principle of meeting the customer's need through a one-by-one continuous flow process with built-in quality indicators and the elimination of system waste.

Another American influence on Toyota was W. Edwards Deming, the American quality pioneer. He defined a "customer" both internally and externally. "Each person or step in a production line or business process was to be treated as a 'customer' and to be supplied with exactly what was needed, at the exact time needed."[1] This view incorporates Toyota's work ethic of demonstrating respect to those who do the work, thus encouraging them to be successful. Another crucial idea adopted from Deming was "a systematic approach to problem solving," referred to as kaizen or continuous improvement, which was intended to sustain TPS daily and to incorporate the frontline staff in decision making.[1]

In the 1960s, Toyota began sharing its successful business practice with its suppliers, creating a "lean enterprise." It was not until the global recession caused by the oil crisis of 1973 that other manufacturing industries in Japan took notice of Toyota. During this time, Toyota did not suffer the great losses of other companies and was asked by the Japanese government to hold seminars on TPS.[1]

American businesses were not exposed to the Toyota Production System until 1982. This exposure was accomplished through a joint venture decision by Eiji Toyoda (chairman) and Shoichiro Toyoda (president) and General Motors, establishing the New United Motor Manufacturing in Fremont, California.[1] Toyota's intention was freely and honestly to share TPS with competitors, whom the company openly acknowledged as contributors to the system of lean production. In a meeting in Japan with Philip Caldwell, the head of Ford Motor Company, Eiji Toyoda stated that, "There is no secret to how we learned what we do, Mr. Caldwell. We learned it at the Rouge."[3] To expand Toyota's teachings to United States industries, the Toyota Supplier Support Center was created in 1992 to provide working TPS models to various plants.[1]

The term "lean production" was introduced in the 1990s by the authors of the book *The Machine That Changed the World,* a Massachusetts Institute of Technology Auto Industry Program that documented what Toyota had discovered decades earlier: "shortening lead time by eliminating waste in each step of a process leads to best quality and lowest cost, while improving safety and morale."[1] It had taken Toyota 40 years to develop its model for producing high-quality cars at low cost, with short lead-time and allowance for broad-based production flexibility. Its dominance of the industry has been unmatched by any other automobile company.

HOW DID TOYOTA DO IT?

Over the last 40 years, Toyota has continued to strive toward the elimination of waste—the heart of TPS—by following a one-by-one continuous flow process. The system is designed to highlight problems in real time, where the work is performed, and solve them to root cause. Many companies have tried to implement this systematic approach to problem solving, but most are unsuccessful. Many emulators focus on the tools used in TPS instead of its basic principles. Moreover, our current "blame culture" is not conducive to this type of system redesign and problem solving. We opt to blame a person and tell him or her to "work harder," rather than to determine the root cause of a problem. A problem often is the result of system-design issues and could be produced by anyone performing the same task.

System errors occur in every industry, and it may be the strategy for addressing them that is critical to success. Solving problems to root cause ensures that they will not recur in a given manner in the future. How does Toyota do it? The question of Toyota's success was addressed in an article by Spear and Bowen,[4] "Decoding the DNA of the Toyota Production System." The authors discovered "unspoken rules that give Toyota its competitive edge." They write, "The system grew naturally out of the workings of the company over five decades . . . it has never been written down and Toyota's workers often are not able to articulate it."[4]

The connection between people and their work is crucial to the success of this process. Leadership support and the involvement of the frontline employee are integral parts of lean production. Spears and Bowen define these connections as the "Four Rules." The first three rules emphasize the design of work. "Rule #1: All work should be highly specified as to content, sequence, timing and outcome. Rule #2: Every customer–supplier connection must be direct and there must be an unambiguous yes-or-no way to send requests and receive responses. Rule #3: The pathway for every product and service must be simple and direct."[4] Rule #4 of the "Four Rules" stresses improvement: "Any improvements must be made in accordance with the scientific method, under the guidance of a teacher, at the lowest possible level in the organization."[4]

Also integral to the TPS model is that "all the rules require that activities, connections, and flow paths have built-in tests to signal problems automatically. It is the continual response to problems that makes this seemingly rigid system so flexible and adaptable to changing circumstances."[4] In Toyota plants, employees are encouraged to announce problems to a team leader by pulling an andon cord, which signals by sound and color where a problem is; acknowledging problems creates the opportunity for improvement. By "lowering the water level in the river to expose all the rocks, [one can] chip away at all the problems."[2] The team leader is used as a real-time problem-solving resource, with one team leader assigned to every four to five team members. On average, an employee pulls the andon cord 12 times per shift.[5] When the team leader solves the problem, the assembly line continues. The line is stopped when the problem cannot be immediately resolved. The problem is then investigated by using the "five whys" to solve it to its root cause. By contrast, our culture traditionally creates "work-arounds" that allow work to continue but do not identify or fully investigate the problem. As a result, problems tend to recur.

A recent book by Jeffrey K. Liker, *The Toyota Way: 14 Management Principles from the World's Greatest Manufacturer,* expands on the success of TPS. "TPS is the most systematic and highly developed example of what the principles of the Toyota Way can accomplish. The Toyota Way consists of the foundational principles of the Toyota culture, which allow TPS to function so effectively."[1] The President of Toyota, Fujio Cho, stated in the 2001 Toyota Way document that "Since Toyota's founding we have adhered to the core principles of contributing to society through the practice of manufacturing high-quality products and services. Our business practices and activities based on this core principle created values, beliefs, and business methods that over the years have become a source of competitive advantage. These are the managerial values and business methods that are known collectively as the Toyota Way."[1]

The Toyota Way is organized into four general categories: "(1) Long-Term Philosophy, (2) The Right Process Will Produce the Right Results, (3) Add Value to the Organization by Developing Your People, and (4) Continuously Solving Root Problems Drives Organizational Learning."[1] The principles associated with each of these categories are listed in Box 1.[1] An examination of these principles clarifies why many companies have been unsuccessful in implementing TPS. Toyota's success is built on its culture of determination, patience, employee involvement, and problem solving by

Box 1. The 14 Toyota Way principles.

Category 1: Long-term philosophy
  Principle 1: Base your management decisions on a long-term philosophy, even at the expense of short-term financial goals.

Category 2: The right process will produce the right results
  Principle 2: Create continuous process flow to bring problems to the surface.
  Principle 3: Use "pull" systems to avoid overproduction.
  Principle 4: Level out the workload (heijunka). (Work like the tortoise, not the hare.)
  Principle 5: Build a culture of stopping to fix problems, to get quality right the first time.
  Principle 6: Standardized tasks are the foundation for continuous improvement and employee empowerment.
  Principle 7: Use visual control so no problems are hidden.
  Principle 8: Use only reliable, thoroughly tested technology that serves your people and processes.

Category 3: Add value to the organization by developing your people and partners
  Principle 9: Grow leaders who thoroughly understand the work, live the philosophy, and teach it to others.
  Principle 10: Develop exceptional people and teams who follow your company's philosophy.
  Principle 11: Respect your extended network of partners and suppliers by challenging them and helping them improve.

Category 4: Continuously solving root problems drives organizational learning
  Principle 12: Go and see for yourself to thoroughly understand the situation (genchi genbutsu).
  Principle 13: Make decisions slowly by consensus, thoroughly considering all options; implement decisions rapidly (nemawashi).
  Principle 14: Become a learning organization through relentless reflection (hansei) and continuous improvement (kaizen).

Source: Adapted from J. K. Liker, The Toyota Way: 14 Management Principles from the World's Greatest Manufacturer (New York: McGraw-Hill, 2004): 37–41.

the scientific method. Many other industries are unable to commit to long-term plans and lack the resources for root cause problem solving; hence they tend to adopt specific tools of TPS and not the entire system.

CAN "LEAN" HELP THE HEALTHCARE SYSTEM?

The rising costs, decreasing reimbursements, malpractice suits, and shortage and dissatisfaction of healthcare professionals have all contributed to the troubling state of our healthcare system. Questions about the quality of healthcare were brought to the forefront by the staggering statistics in the Institute of Medicine's (IOM) report "To Err Is Human: Building a Safer Health System."[6] The IOM found medical errors (defined as the failure of a planned action to be completed or use of the wrong plan to achieve an aim) to be the "eighth leading cause of death," surpassing deaths from motor vehicle accidents, breast cancer, and AIDS.

In Pittsburgh, there has been a growing initiative to address medical errors. The Pittsburgh Regional Health Care Initiative (PRHI) was formed in 1997 to address the economic and patient safety issues of healthcare in southwestern Pennsylvania, where "healthcare is the largest economic sector, employing one in eight workers and conducting more than $7.2 billion in business."[7] Founded by Paul O'Neill, former U.S. Treasury Secretary and Alcoa Chairman, and Karen Wolk Feinstein, PhD, President of the Jewish Healthcare Foundation, with the mission of providing programs aimed at perfect patient care, PRHI is an alliance of "hundreds of clinicians, 42 hospitals, four major insurers, dozens of major and small business healthcare purchasers, corporate and civic leaders, and elected officials."[7] The Initiative's "patient-centered goals include zero medication errors, zero healthcare-acquired (nosocomial) infections, [and] perfect clinical outcomes, as measured by complications, readmissions, and other patient outcomes, specifically in coronary artery bypass graft surgery and chronic conditions (depression and diabetes)."[7] To accomplish these goals, PRHI has incorporated principles from industrial lean production models, including TPS and

Pittsburgh's Alcoa Business System, to design a model for healthcare called the Perfecting Patient Care (PPC) System.[8] The fundamental principles of the organization are "respect and dignity for everyone, the opportunity for healthcare workers to succeed in doing meaningful work and to have it acknowledged, neutral collaboration among all stakeholders, and improvement based on scientific methods, applied to every patient every day."[7] PRHI offers year-round courses to the public to teach and share the knowledge of the PPC System within the region.

Through grants from the Jewish Healthcare Foundation, the Agency for Health Care Research and Quality, and the University of Pittsburgh School of Medicine, the authors' pathology laboratory chose to adopt the principles of lean production (or the PPC System) to address pathology errors. The implementation of a lean production method begins with leadership support. Leadership throughout the organization, from top administration to frontline supervision, needs to understand and demonstrate approval for the process. Otherwise, implementation will most likely fail. In the authors' organization, implementation began in September 2003 when the laboratory obtained support from the hospital CEO, vice presidents, president, and vice president of the medical staff and developed an education plan for the pathology administration and staff. Education methods included both in-house training sessions and attendance of sessions taught by the PRHI.

Initially, these teachings may be difficult to apply to healthcare because they have manufacturing biases whose relevance may not be apparent. The natural and immediate reaction from some of our laboratory staff was resistance: "We don't make cars here. We work with patient specimens." Several were concerned about the comparison of their work to an industrial process, feeling as if it diminished or simplified their jobs. "You can't apply [the model of] a manufacturing company to our work. Our work is more complicated." Other staff members liked the idea of eliminating waste and improving their work but had doubts that principles from manufacturing could be the answer. Still others expressed their frustration with the current state of the healthcare system and welcomed the idea of trying "anything new" and the opportunity to be part of the change. Everyone wants to take pride in his or her work and achieve success.

ANATOMIC PATHOLOGY
LEARNING LINE

To begin establishing what is referred to as a learning line for implementation of a lean production method, one must document the current workflow condition. The role of the team leader (real-time problem solver) for a learning line begins immediately. The leader assures the trust and confidence of the staff involved in implementation through daily teachings and by engaging the staff in generating ideas and sharing information about how they do their work. Observation drawings, a pictorial documentation of workflow pathways, are an important tool adopted from the PPC System.[9] Assumptions about how work is done or should be done often differ from reality. By observing how work is actually performed, one may establish a solid baseline from which to begin workflow and process improvements.

The observation process entails several elements, including demonstrating respect for those one observes. PRHI has established the following recommended Observation Guidelines: "(1) Explain what you are observing to the person being observed and that you are interested in learning from them through observation. They are the teachers of the current condition and you will be observing to learn. (2) Try not to be obtrusive and not to modify the process you are trying to observe. (3) Do not ask 'why' and limit questions. These may be asked at the completion of the observation so as not to interfere. (4) At the end of the observation, thank the person you observed."[9] Although the observation process seems straightforward, this may be a difficult exercise to perform. Staff members will naturally feel uncomfortable performing their work when they know someone is watching their every move and perhaps timing them. In the authors' experience, staff often wanted to point out, "This isn't a normal day" or "This is an unusual circumstance" when they believed the observer might gain a negative impression. It is important to demonstrate sensitivity during these sessions. Other staff members were anxious to explain their work in detail, which was helpful in establishing a comfort level.

To convey the team leader's support for staff work improvement, multiple observations were performed and time was spent talking with the frontline staff. Through data collection and observation drawings, the current condition of the authors' anatomic pathology department was documented, beginning with specimen receipt and ending with the generation of a report to clinicians (Figure D.1). A current condition drawing represents the workflow pathway, drawn according to customer/supplier relationships. The connections between the customer making the request (need) and the supplier meeting the need, as well as how the individual worker performs his or her work (activities), define a pathway.

The authors' anatomic pathology pathway is initiated upon receipt of a specimen from one of their customers (operating room, in-house patients, or outpatient clinics) in the gross room. Here the specimen is appropriately accessioned, grossly examined, and sectioned, with the tissue placed in colored plastic cassettes and the cassettes placed in a rack for the overnight tissue processing machines. The gross room is the supplier of the next step in surgical specimen processing, the histology lab. Histology processes the cassettes the following morning by embedding the tissue in wax and cutting thin pieces of tissue to be stained and placed on a glass slide. The histology lab is the supplier of the pathologist, who reviews the slide and provides a diagnosis for transcription. Transcription then becomes the customer of the pathologist, transcribing the report for the ordering physician. The physician is the supplier of the patient, the ultimate customer.

Included in the current condition drawings are problems, designated as inverted clouds, that have occurred or are system designs to be addressed using the principles of lean. Problems may range from ones as simple as a staff member asking a coworker for a pen and having to search for a supply to more serious ones affecting patient care. Identifying problems is a challenging part of this process. As mentioned earlier, medical culture has adopted the practice of "work-arounds," in which we attempt to solve a problem ourselves and, often without realizing it, create additional steps as a Band-Aid to the problem. Because they do not entail investigating the problem to its root cause, these "work-arounds" become a form of waste in the system. However, it is not easy for workers to acknowledge this extra waste and identify it as a problem. This situation provides another example of the role of the team leader. By working daily with the

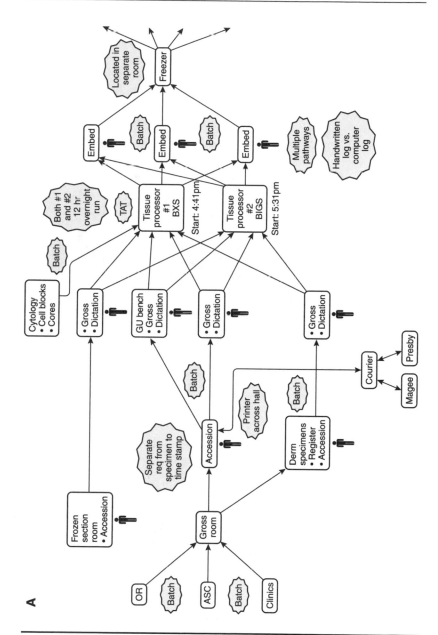

Figure D.1 UPMC Shadyside Anatomic Pathology Laboratory—
current condition.

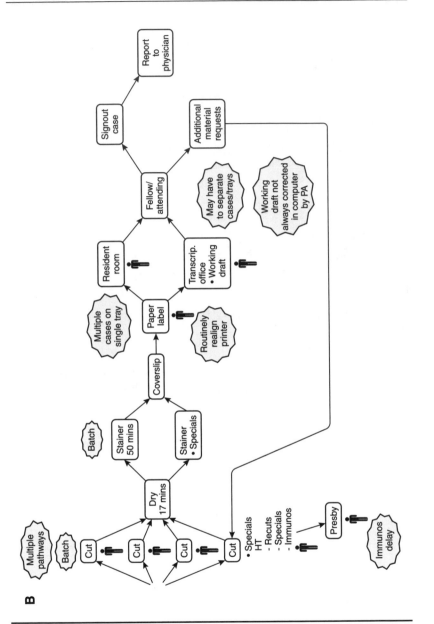

Figure D.1 *Continued.*

staff to teach lean principles and their application to work practices, the leader enables staff to begin identifying the waste in their own work.

Once the current condition has been documented, research focuses on determining the ideal. According to the basic principles of lean, the goals to strive toward are one-by-one and continuous flow work design. Spear and Bowen[4] describe "the notion of the ideal" as essential to understanding TPS. The response to customer need must embody six characteristics: on demand, defect-free, one-by-one, waste-free, immediate, and safe (physically, emotionally, professionally).[4] In pathology, the ultimate goal is to provide appropriate and accurate information about a patient's specimen to a clinician for quality patient care. Ideally, this is accomplished with zero pathology errors (that is, assignments of a diagnosis that does not represent the true nature of disease or nondisease in a patient, as a result of either interpretive or reporting errors). The idea of zero pathology errors may seem unrealistic, but if we do not continually strive toward this theoretic limit, how will we know what is possible? Human potential is limitless—a philosophy practiced successfully by Toyota. As noted previously, everyone wants to succeed at his or her job, though poor system designs often prevent this success.

Demand data are also collected to enhance understanding of the current condition. Demand data (Tables D.1 and D.2) reflect customer need. The mix, volume, and timing of the demand must be understood first (that is, How much of what is needed when?). The next question is "What does it take to make one to perfection?" Mix and volume refer to the type and amount of work.

Table D.1 Anatomic pathology demand data.

Mix	Volume (%)
Biopsy specimens	13
Skin specimens	24
Surgical ("large") specimens	63

Table D.2   Anatomic pathology demand data.

Timing	
Specimens received from	**Pickup times**
OR	8:00 AM, 10:00 AM, 11:00 AM, 1:00 PM, 2:15 PM
ASC	8:00 AM, 10:00 AM, 11:00 AM, 1:00 PM
Clinics	9:00 AM, 9:20 AM, 10:50 AM, 12:15 PM, 12:30 PM, 2:40 PM

For example, the authors' anatomic pathology laboratory receives specimens from the operating room and various physicians' offices and departments. The types of specimens received and processed include soft tissue, bone, prostate, kidney, breast, biopsies, skin, and cytology cell blocks (63 percent surgical specimens, 24 percent skin specimens, 12 percent biopsy specimens, and one percent cytology cell blocks). Each of these types of specimens requires different work to be performed. Timing refers to the frequency of each type of work. The laboratory has both daily scheduled and unscheduled specimen pickups. Fluctuations in volume of certain types of specimens occur daily or weekly.

Once one has established the current condition through work-flow observation, problem identification, and collection of demand data, one may determine the direction and possibilities for improving workflow design. The authors' intention was to establish an anatomic pathology learning line and design a one-by-one continuous flow process. Histology, with its inherent "assembly line" workflow design, was designated as the first section of the department to establish this line. Starting with the central portion of the anatomic pathology pathway, one may affect change at both ends of the pathology process.

Once the decision was made to begin in histology, administrative support from histology supervision and the lead histotechnologist was generated. Staff were presented with the current condition and a plan to apply the principles of lean production to improve workflow design and strive toward zero pathology errors. Concentrated teaching began among the team leader, the TPS teacher, and histology staff. Focused observation documented the specific current condition pathway of histology (Figure D.2). This observation focused on

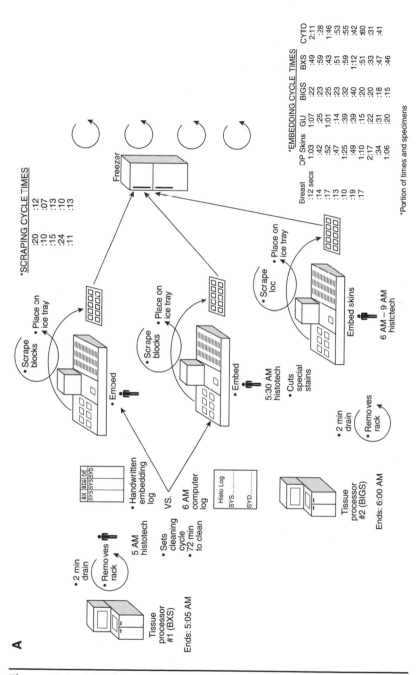

Figure D.2 Histology—current condition (includes cycle times for each task).

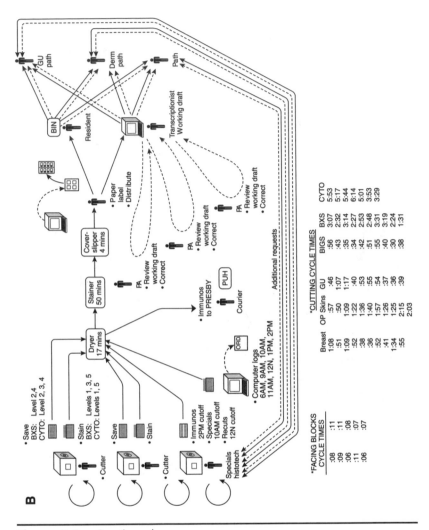

Figure D.2 *Continued.*

how tasks were performed, the amount of time it took to perform each task, how tasks were connected to accomplish work, and problems that arose during the course of work.

Cycle-time data were collected on each histotechnologist for each job task, as was instrumentation timing in the pathway. Cycle time is the time it takes to perform the work activities of one work element (for example, embedding or cutting).[2] For example, the "average" cycle time to embed biopsies was 57 seconds; for cutting, it was 192 seconds, more than triple the amount of time to embed. This discrepancy created an unbalanced workflow, which was evaluated to determine whether any of the cutting tasks could be separated and accomplished at another workstation. For instance, slides could be premade by the embedder to save time for the cutter. This measure is referred to as work balancing, or ensuring that job tasks performed at each station have closer cycle times to maintain balance in the work elements of the pathway. Without work balancing, inventory will build up between work processes. The concept of continuous flow implies that a tissue moves from one work process to the next, with no wasted time waiting in the production line.

Following observational data collection, the histology staff and supervisors of anatomic pathology participated in a lean exercise. Staff were taught the principles of the lean production method through a hands-on exercise in which they mimicked a manufacturing assembly line. The exercise generated mixed reactions from the staff, including resistance to the notion of applying this method to laboratory work, anxiety that the process might eliminate positions, and enthusiasm about trying something different. Leadership was able to address the concerns about position elimination by stressing that this was not the aim of the process.

THE 5S PROCESS

To begin winning the "hearts and minds" of the staff to these new principles, a kaizen—or system improvement—called 5S was initiated. The objective of this process was to clean up and improve the work environment. The process began with a red-tagging session in which the staff placed a red label on any products or equipment they no longer used. All red-tagged items were removed from the laboratory, and the staff decided whether items could be sold, given to another department, or discarded (Figure D.3). The histotechnologists enjoyed this process, because they had wanted to "get rid of the junk" but had not had time to do so. Once the excess was removed, determinations regarding workflow improvements were made using 5S. "5S" refers to the different steps of this process: sort (Japanese seiri, meaning to organize); set in order (seiton, orderliness); shine

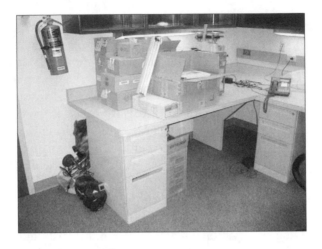

Figure D.3 Portion of items from red-tagging for 5S.

(seiso, cleanliness); standardize (seiketsu, standardized cleanup); and sustain (shitsuke, discipline to maintain this process).[9] To demonstrate the effectiveness of this process, one particular "cell" of the laboratory, the special stain section (Figure D.4), was targeted for redesign, so that only products, supplies, and equipment needed to perform these stains were in the cell.

On one evening, a team consisting of nine members from PRHI, the Clinical Design Team of Shadyside Hospital (which began using the PPC System in 1998 for patient care improvements), the chief and director of Shadyside Pathology, the team leader, the TPS teacher, and additional pathology supervisory staff cleaned the histology laboratory from top to bottom (Figure D.5). From scouring sinks to scrubbing floors and drawers, the team successfully "5S'ed" the laboratory and began creating a visual management atmosphere by tagging drawers to indicate where products were stored (Figure D.6). The next morning, the histotechnologists were pleasantly surprised by the appearance of their lab and the show of support from the staff who accomplished it.

Additional visual management improvements were made in the designated special stain cell by the histotechnologists. These included labeling the outside of the stain and dye cabinets with both

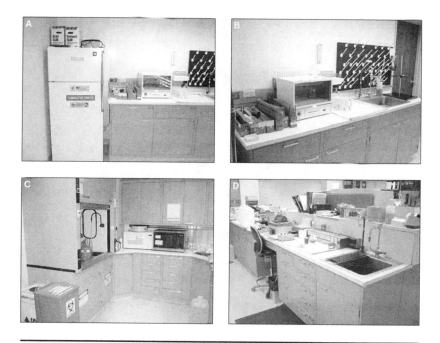

Figure D.4 (*A–D*) Special staining cell before 5S.

pictures and terms to represent what was on the shelf directly behind the cabinet door and color-coding the special stain baskets according to end-color result of each stain (Figure D.7).

During this time, process improvements were also made to address the excess inventory in histology. The histotechnologist responsible for the routine ordering process was instrumental in designing a new replenishment system. This design was accomplished through the use of kanban cards, adopted from TPS.[2] Each product was tagged with a kanban card that included all the information necessary to reorder it: product name, reorder quantity, and trigger point. The trigger point indicated where the card needed to be placed when the product was restocked. This point was determined by calculating the amount of product routinely used and how many days from the ordering date it took to receive the product. The system was based on the three different ordering processes of the laboratory. Products with blue cards, for example, were to be ordered

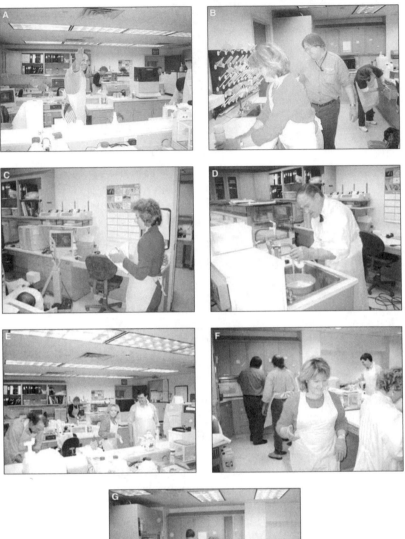

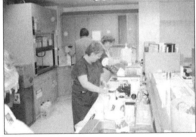

Figure D.5 *(A–G)* 5S group process.

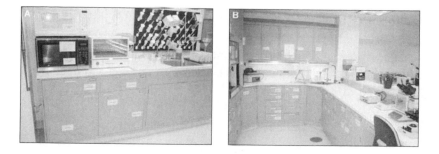

Figure D.6 (*A,B*) Special staining cell after 5S.

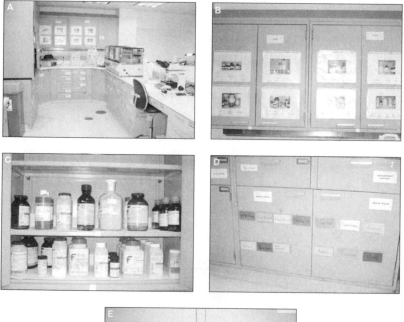

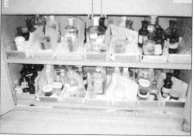

Figure D.7 (*A–E*) Visual management examples.

through a specific vendor, yellow cards were for in-house stock inventory, and pink cards were for the laboratory ordering system. The cards were placed on the product in such a manner as to alert the histotechnologist that it needed to be reordered. When a kanban card was pulled, it was hung on a hook with the corresponding color. It was easy for the histotechnologist to visualize the necessary type of ordering. Once the product was ordered, the card was placed in its corresponding colored bin in the laboratory where products were delivered, so that it could be replaced (Figure D.8). For the ordering histotechnologist, this was a rewarding experience. Her ordering time was cut by at least 50 percent, and she did not have to worry about stocking out or about products not being ordered because someone did not inform her. The system is working well, and the histology laboratory's overstocked inventory has been reduced by approximately 40 percent to 60 percent.

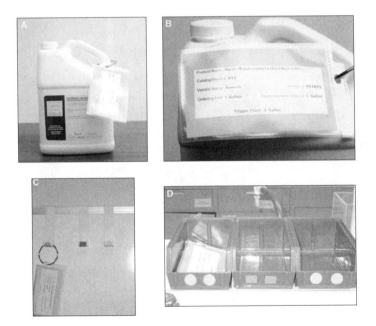

Figure D.8   (*A–D*) Inventory replenishment system (kanban cards). ([A] Courtesy of Anatech Ltd., Battle Creek, Michigan; with permission.)

CONTINUOUS FLOW

The next phase of the authors' implementation was to create a continuous workflow. To create this type of work practice, one must eliminate waste or non-value-added work. Taiichi Ohno[2] describes seven different forms of waste: overproduction, excess movement, excess waiting time, excess inventory, processing waste, transportation waste, and manufacture of defective products. In the laboratory, there are many examples of these forms of waste. For example, laboratory personnel are accustomed to working with large batch sizes, working separately from the next workstation in the process, and having excess inventory on hand.

The waste arising from batching and separation of the different workstations needed to accomplish a process was apparent in the authors' histology department. The original layout of the histology laboratory was as follows: a side room contained three machines for the embedding of tissue and a separate room with five microtomes for the cutting of tissue (Figure D.9). Up to three histotechnologists could be performing the task of embedding at once, while one histotechnologist began cutting. Because the embedders supplied the large number of blocks to be cut, it was necessary to place the blocks on an ice tray in a freezer to keep them cold until a cutter could get to them. This procedure created a large batch of trays for the cutting process. The embedders would pursue their work to completion, then assist with the cutting process. This practice of mass-producing one task, then moving to the next is not unusual and has most likely been practiced for years in many histology laboratories. It does, however, highlight the opportunity to use lean production practices to eliminate these types of system-design waste and to improve pathology practice. When one designs a continuous flow process, one establishes a direct connection between work tasks: the embedder becomes the supplier to the customer, the cutter. To create this direct line of communication in the authors' laboratory, an embedding machine was moved to a counter in the cutting area, and the remainder of the process (primarily instrumentation) was rearranged in order of operation. The end result was a "U-shaped" cell (Figure D.10). This arrangement was a dramatic change for the histotechnologists, who naturally doubted that it would work. The fact that they were willing

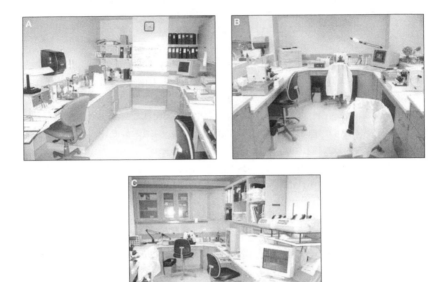

Figure D.9 Histology department layout. (*A*) Embedding room. (*B,C*) Cutting areas.

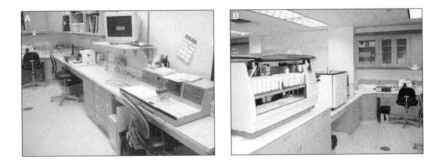

Figure D.10 (*A,B*) Continuous flow.

to try and did not completely resist this experiment in the lean principles was a critical step in the implementation process.

Once the new cell was created, reducing the batch sizes to create a continuous flow and to help prevent the potential for error became an objective. Although the cell had been physically arranged in a continuous flow design, the tendency of the histotechnologists was still to batch-produce at each workstation. Defining and designing the necessary direct connection between the embedder and the cutter required the input of the histotechnologists, those who do the work, under the guidance of the team leader and teacher using the principles of lean. The ideas of not batch-processing and of handing work directly to the cutter (rather than putting trays in the freezer) were significant challenges, because this was unlike any practice the histotechnologists had experienced.

The process began with small experiments intended to demonstrate the true nature of how work is done: one by one; one block, one slide at a time. Answering the question "What is one?" was also challenging. In the gross room, for instance, "one" most likely refers to one patient or one accession number, which could have multiple specimens. In histology, work is performed on tissue blocks to produce slides. When the team had examined the work done on each type of specimen processed, the answer to "What is one?" became a slide. From this determination, it was decided that a maximum of 20 slides (the number that completely filled a slide rack) would be made by the cutter, then passed through the remainder of the process. (This number was chosen for practicality, because of the instrumentation limitation of the stainer.) Hence the embedder (supplier) would send at one time to the cutter (customer) only enough blocks to produce a maximum of 20 slides. This limitation dramatically changed the embedder's work practice. The histotechnologists were being asked to embed only a designated number of blocks—then, once those blocks were appropriately cold, to stop embedding, scrape them, and pass them to the cutter. The cutter previously took her work from the freezer; her work consisted of an ice tray full of blocks, and she filled multiple slide racks before moving them through the process.

Table D.3 illustrates this application of lean production to the reduction of batch sizes, eventually to one, by explaining the amount of work performed on each specimen type. For biopsy specimens,

Table D.3 Histology specimen requirements.

Specimen	No. of slides made	No. of slides stained	No. of slides saved
Biopsy specimens	5	3	2
Cytology cell block	5	2	3
Skin specimens	2	2	0
Surgical ("large") specimens	1	1	0

five slides are made, three are stained, and two are saved for future additional stain requests. These figures mean that the embedder makes and passes six biopsy blocks to the cutter, who makes a total of 18 slides, then sends the slide rack to the dryer to continue the process. If the blocks are from skin specimens, 10 blocks can be made for the cutter to produce 20 slides, and if the blocks are from "large" specimens (for example, tissue sections from a mastectomy), 20 blocks make 20 slides. After many experiments over time, the histotechnologists began developing a comfort level with this new type of production. The work was still not at the ideal state of continuous flow, in which one specimen was embedded at a time and passed directly to the cutter, who made the appropriate number of slides and passed them through the rest of the process. The histotechnologists were, however, able to appreciate that overproduction was not making their work easier or faster; indeed, it had added more stress.

Another important aspect of winning the "hearts and minds" of the staff involved in this lean process was enabling them to recognize the importance of their work. Everyone wants to be successful in his or her job, but often workers are so far removed from their customer that they lack this sense of accomplishment. Pathology is a good example. The diagnosis provided to the clinician by the pathologist has a direct impact on a patient's care. Many are not aware of the complex process needed to provide the most accurate information to the physician. To help bring this end result of their work into perspective for the histotechnologists, a connection was made directly to the patient. The difference was in the thinking: a block is a patient, and work should be performed on that patient continuously to provide an "answer" to him or her as rapidly as possible. To highlight this principle, a bladder specimen was followed through the pathology pathway from its removal from the patient in the operating room to the autofaxing of a report to the physician (Figure D.11). The amount of work actually performed on the specimen (indicated by slashes) was approximately 14 hours, whereas the amount of time the specimen was at rest (open spaces) was approximately 87 hours, including the weekend. This is not unusual pathology practice, and it demonstrates the need to improve our system to decrease the time between collection of a patient specimen and rendering of a diagnosis.

The histotechnologists have demonstrated many successes of adopting a lean process; however, there are still many challenges ahead. As histology approaches the ideal, changes will need to occur at both ends of the pathology pathway. The gross room, for example, should consistently produce tissue blocks with only the amount of (defect-free) tissue necessary for histology to perform its work. Pathologists should be able to sign out cases continuously as they are being produced from histology. At this point, the improvements in the histology pathway have not made significant changes in the overall report turnaround time, but once the gross room and pathology sign-out work elements are incorporated, the authors expect that this time will be significantly reduced.

Currently, the histotechnologists have adopted the practice of smaller batch sizes and continue to work on a true one-by-one processing system. Effective problem solving to root cause will assist in reaching this goal. Once a problem is identified, the team leader and staff work together to identify its cause and find a resolution. PRHI teaches the use of a tool called a Problem Solving A3 (named for the size of paper used to document the problem) to help guide this process.[9] The paper is divided into four quadrants: (1) the background of the process and problem that arose, (2) answers to the "five whys" to determine the root cause of the problem, (3) determination of the target condition in which the problem does not recur, and (4) the action plan or experiments using the scientific method that clearly define the who, what, when, where, and how of the experiment (Table D.4). The authors' histology lab recently encountered a problem that

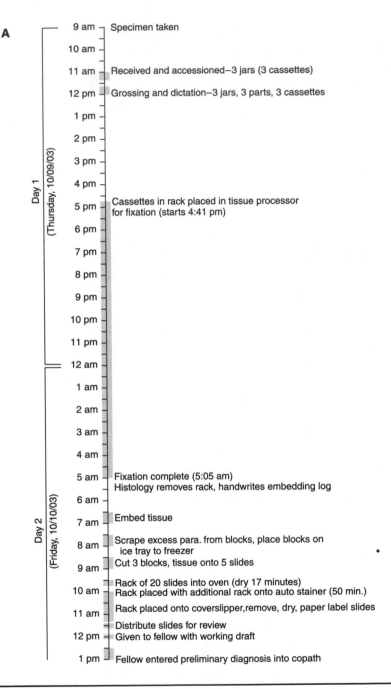

A

Day 1 (Thursday, 10/09/03)

9 am — Specimen taken

10 am —

11 am — Received and accessioned–3 jars (3 cassettes)

12 pm — Grossing and dictation–3 jars, 3 parts, 3 cassettes

1 pm —

2 pm —

3 pm —

4 pm —

5 pm — Cassettes in rack placed in tissue processor for fixation (starts 4:41 pm)

6 pm —

7 pm —

8 pm —

9 pm —

10 pm —

11 pm —

Day 2 (Friday, 10/10/03)

12 am —

1 am —

2 am —

3 am —

4 am —

5 am — Fixation complete (5:05 am)
Histology removes rack, handwrites embedding log

6 am —

7 am — Embed tissue

8 am — Scrape excess para. from blocks, place blocks on ice tray to freezer

9 am — Cut 3 blocks, tissue onto 5 slides

10 am — Rack of 20 slides into oven (dry 17 minutes)
Rack placed with additional rack onto auto stainer (50 min.)

11 am — Rack placed onto coverslipper,remove, dry, paper label slides

Distribute slides for review

12 pm — Given to fellow with working draft

1 pm — Fellow entered preliminary diagnosis into copath

Figure D.11   Pathology pathway: bladder specimen example. *(Continued)*

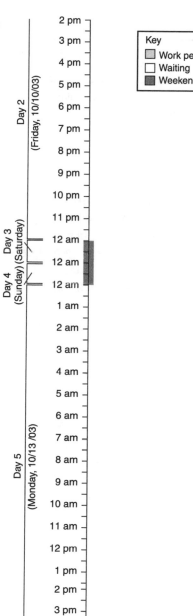

B

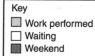

Figure D.11 *(Continued.)*

Table D.4 Problem solving A3.

(1) Background; current condition	(3) Target condition
(2) Problem defined	(4) Action plan

Adapted from Pittsburgh Regional Healthcare Initiative. Perfecting Patient Care System educational materials.

clearly demonstrated the value of solving to the root cause, rather than accepting a superficial solution.

One day, the histotechnologist responsible for cutting slides for immunohistochemistry studies received a computer-generated block order for recuts and additional slides. When she retrieved the block, she noted a scant amount of tissue remaining and observed the number three written on the side of the cassette, indicating the number of pieces originally embedded in the block. She made a notation on the order sheet, "Block very thin before cut immunos," and proceeded to complete the order. Two days later, she received the same request as before, this time with a notation by the pathologist: "*Wrong* block cut!!!" Concerned about and upset by this possible error, the histotechnologist repulled the block and alerted a coworker to the problem. Much time was spent examining other blocks in consecutive order to try to determine how the original slides looked so different from the reprocessed slides. A solution was not determined until later in the day, when the coworker assisting on the case happened to remember a block that had "chunked out" on her microtome a few days earlier. When this accident occurred, the coworker retrieved the remaining specimen from her water bath; thus tissue was available that matched the original slides reviewed by the pathologist. Until this point, the immunohistochemical histotechnologist did not have resolution, and she indicated that she felt "her professionalism was being called into question."

The cause of the scant amount of tissue in the block was actually an instrumentation problem. By standard design, there are two latches in close proximity to each other on the microtome: one to unlock and replace the cutting blade and one to adjust the cutting angle (Figure D.12). On the day of the incident, the histotechnologist had changed her blade and was unaware that the latch for the

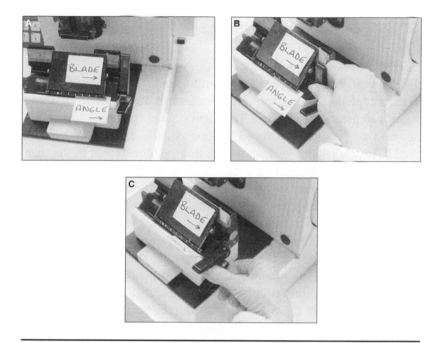

Figure D.12   (*A–C*) Example of root cause analysis. Close proximity of latches enables blade angle to change from routine cutting angle of 10° to 0°.

blade angle had shifted. When she resumed cutting, the blade made a deep cut, resulting in the loss of tissue. Measures are currently being taken to help prevent this from happening again. A rubber stopper is being placed between the two latches to reduce the likelihood of displacing the blade angle.

This story highlights many of the problems we face in healthcare. Had this problem not been solved to its true root cause, the mechanical problem might not have been addressed, and any of the histotechnologists using that microtome could have had the same unfortunate accident. The pathologist, as well as the immunohistochemical histotechnologist herself, would have questioned her professionalism in the future. The pathologist's statement "*Wrong* block cut!!!" immediately created a defensive atmosphere. Placing the blame on a person may be detrimental to finding a solution and, ultimately, to improving the system.

SUMMARY

The current state of our healthcare system calls for dramatic changes. In their pathology department, the authors believe these changes may be accomplished by accepting the long-term commitment of applying a lean production system. The ideal state of zero pathology errors is one that should be pursued by consistently asking, "Why can't we?" The philosophy of lean production systems began in the manufacturing industry: "All we are doing is looking at the time from the moment the customer gives us an order to the point when we collect the cash. And we are reducing that time line by removing non-value-added wastes."[2] The ultimate goals in pathology and overall health care are not so different. The authors' intention is to provide the patient (customer) with the most accurate diagnostic information in a timely and efficient manner. Their lead histotechnologist recently summarized this philosophy: she indicated that she felt she could sleep better at night knowing she truly did the best job she could. Her chances of making an error (in cutting or labeling) were dramatically decreased in the one-by-one continuous flow work process compared with previous practices. By designing a system that enables employees to be successful in meeting customer demand, and by empowering the frontline staff in the development and problem-solving processes, one can meet the challenges of eliminating waste and build an improved, efficient system.

Appendix E
Going Lean in Health Care

This paper is based on presentations made by the following experts during an IHI Calls to Action Series in January and February 2005:
James P. Womack, PhD: *Founder and President, Lean Enterprise Institute*
Arthur P. Byrne, MBA: *Operating Partner, JW Childs Associates LLC*
Orest J. Fiume, MS: *Co-author, "Real Numbers: Management Accounting in a Lean Organization"*
Gary S. Kaplan, MD, FACP, FACMPE: *Chairman and CEO, Virginia Mason Medical Center*
John Toussaint, MD: *President and CEO, ThedaCare, Inc.*

Editor: Diane Miller, MBA: *Director, IHI*

EXECUTIVE SUMMARY

Lean management principles have been used effectively in manufacturing companies for decades, particularly in Japan. The Institute for Healthcare Improvement believes that lean principles can be—indeed, already are being—successfully applied to the delivery of health care.

Lean thinking begins with driving out waste so that all work adds value and serves the customer's needs. Identifying value-added and non-value-added steps in every process is the beginning of the journey toward lean operations.

In order for lean principles to take root, leaders must first work to create an organizational culture that is receptive to lean thinking. The commitment to lean must start at the very top of the organization, and all staff should be involved in helping to redesign processes to improve flow and reduce waste.

Although health care differs in many ways from manufacturing, there are also surprising similarities: Whether building a car or providing health care for a patient, workers must rely on multiple, complex processes to accomplish their tasks and provide value to the customer or patient. Waste—of money, time, supplies, or good will—decreases value.

Examples in this paper of lean thinking in health care demonstrate that, when applied rigorously and throughout an entire organization, lean principles can have a positive impact on productivity, cost, quality, and timely delivery of services.

INTRODUCTION

The concept called "lean management" or "lean thinking" is most commonly associated with Japanese manufacturing, particularly the Toyota Production System (TPS). Much of the TPS way of thinking is based on the work of quality guru W. Edwards Deming, who taught, among other things, that managers should stop depending on mass inspection to achieve quality and, instead, focus on improving the production process and building quality into the product in the first place.

So what is meant by "lean thinking"? Simply put, lean means using less to do more.

Lean thinking is not typically associated with health care, where waste—of time, money, supplies, and good will—is a common problem. But the principles of lean management can, in fact, work in health care in much the same way they do in other industries. This paper presents a brief overview of lean management principles, and provides examples of two health care organizations that are successfully using lean thinking to streamline processes, reduce cost, and improve quality and timely delivery of products and services.

Lean thinking is not a manufacturing tactic or a cost-reduction program, but a management strategy that is applicable to all organizations because it has to do with improving processes. All organizations—including health care organizations—are composed of a series of processes, or sets of actions intended to create value for those who use or depend on them (customers/patients).

The core idea of lean involves determining the value of any given process by distinguishing value-added steps from non-value-added steps, and eliminating waste (or *muda* in Japanese) so that ultimately every step adds value to the process.

To maximize value and eliminate waste, leaders in health care, as in other organizations, must evaluate processes by accurately specifying the value desired by the user; identifying every step in the process (or "value stream," in the language of lean) and eliminating non-value-added steps; and making value flow from beginning to end based on the pull—the expressed needs—of the customer/patient.

When applied rigorously and throughout an entire organization, lean principles can have a dramatic affect on productivity, cost, and quality. Figure E.1 presents some statistics that testify to the power of lean thinking in industry. There is no *a priori* reason why much of this same effect can't be realized in health care.

Agreement is growing among health care leaders that lean principles can reduce the waste that is pervasive in the US health care system. The Institute for Healthcare Improvement believes that adoption of lean management strategies—while not a simple task—can help health care organizations improve processes and outcomes, reduce cost, and increase satisfaction among patients, providers and staff.

Validated industry averages*	
Direct labor/Productivity improved	45–75%
Cost reduced	25–55%
Throughput/Flow increased	60–90%
Quality (defects/scrap) reduced	50–90%
Inventory reduced	60–90%
Space reduced	35–50%
Lead time reduced	50–90%

*Summarized results, subsequent to a five-year evaluation, from numerous companies (more than 15 aerospace-related). Companies ranged from 1 to >7 years in lean principles application/execution.

Figure E.1   The impact of lean principles in industry.
Source: Virginia Mason Medical Center

THE POWER OF LEAN IN HEALTH CARE

Virginia Mason Medical Center in Seattle, Washington, has been using lean management principles since 2002. By working to eliminate waste, Virginia Mason created more capacity in existing programs and practices so that planned expansions were scrapped, saving significant capital expenses: $1 million for an additional hyperbaric chamber that was no longer needed; $1 to $3 million for endoscopy suites that no longer needed to be relocated; $6 million for new surgery suites that were no longer necessary.

Despite a "no-layoff policy," a key tenet of lean management, staffing trends at Virginia Mason show a decrease in 2003 and 2004, after six years of annual increases in the number of full-time equivalents (FTEs). Using lean principles, staff, providers and patients have continuously improved or redesigned processes to eliminate waste, requiring fewer staff members and less rework, and resulting in better quality. Consequently, as employees retire or leave for other reasons, improved productivity allows for them not to be replaced.

Category	2004 results (after 2 years of "lean")	Metric	Change from 2002
Inventory	$1,350,000	Dollars	Down 53%
Productivity	158	FTEs	36% redeployed to other open positions
Floor space	22,324	Sq. Ft.	Down 41%
Lead time	23,082	Hours	Down 65%
People distance	Traveled 267,793	Feet	Down 44%
Product distance	Traveled 272,262	Feet	Down 72%
Setup time	7,744	Hours	Down 82%

Figure E.2 Results of 175 rapid process improvement weeks at Virginia Mason Medical Center.

Source: Virginia Mason Medical Center

All 5,000 Virginia Mason employees are required to attend an "Introduction to Lean" course, and many have participated in Rapid Process Improvement Weeks (RPIW). RPIWs are intensive week-long sessions in which teams analyze processes and propose, test, and implement improvements. The results from the 175 RPIWs that were conducted from January 2002 through March 2004 are shown in Figure E.2.

How did Virginia Mason achieve these striking results?

KEY CONCEPTS IN LEAN THINKING: LESSONS FROM THE EXPERIENCE IN INDUSTRY

Virginia Mason's achievements were based on lean thinking, the major precepts of which are as follows:

Leadership: Introducing lean thinking in an organization is, in the words of those who have done it, not for the faint of heart. It cannot be done piecemeal, but must be a whole-system strategy. There is no single "silver bullet" solution such as a new computer system or automated equipment that will achieve the same results. And it cannot be done only by middle managers or frontline workers. Those at the very top of the organization must lead it.

Implementing lean thinking requires major change management throughout an entire organization, which can be traumatic and difficult. Strong commitment and inspiring leadership from senior leaders is essential to the success of an effort this challenging. The CEO must be a vocal, visible champion of lean management, create an environment where it is permissible to fail, set stretch goals, and encourage "leaps of faith." A senior management team that is aligned in its vision and understanding of lean is a critical foundation for "going lean."

Culture: A lean culture is the backdrop against which lean tools and techniques are implemented. That culture differs in some significant ways from a traditional culture in business, as well as in health care. Figure E.3 offers some examples.

An organization's culture is the set of values and beliefs that cause people to behave in certain ways. When they behave that way and get the results they expect, it reinforces those values and beliefs. This self-reinforcing cycle creates a culture.

Leaders who wish to change their organizational culture cannot do so by edict. They must intervene and require people to behave differently, allowing them to experience a better set of results. As this process is repeated, a different set of values and beliefs—a new culture—will evolve.

One of the challenges of implementing lean in health care is that it requires people to identify waste in the work in which they are so invested. All workers want to feel their work is valuable, perhaps most especially health care workers. Recognizing that much about their daily tasks is wasteful and does not add value can be difficult for health care professionals. A nurse who is hunting for supplies is doing it to serve the needs of patients. Nurses may not see this as wasted time, and may not stop to wonder why those supplies aren't where they need them every time they need them. But if the supplies were always readily available, the time nurses spend hunting for them would instead be devoted to something more appropriate to their skills and expertise.

To help staff see and embrace the promise of lean, leaders must create a clear vision statement that guides people to make the right choices. They must evaluate the organizational structure and work to flatten it, eliminating hierarchical layers and organizing staff into operational teams based on products or services.

Process: A process is a set of actions or steps, each of which must be accomplished properly in the proper sequence at the proper time to create value for a cus tomer or patient. *Primary* processes serve the external customer (in health care, patients and their families). *Internal* processes serve internal customers/staff in support of the primary process. Primary processes are easier to see, but internal processes are necessary to create value in the primary process.

Compared to other industries, health care has been slow to identify who the customer really is. Because of the complexity of the health care system, internal customers—physicians, hospitals, insurers, government, payers—have often driven processes. It is critically important that value be defined by the primary customer: the patient.

A perfect process creates precisely the right value for the customer. In a perfect process, every step is *valuable* (creates value for the customer), *capable* (produces a good result every time), *available* (produces the desired output, not just the desired quality, every time), *adequate* (does not cause delay), *flexible,* and *linked by continuous flow.* Failure in any of these dimensions produces some type of waste. The Toyota Production System (TPS) identifies seven categories of waste: overproduction, waiting, transporting, processing, inventory, motion, and correction.

A perfect process not only creates value, but it is also satisfying for people to perform, managers to manage, and customers to experience.

GETTING STARTED

To create the perfect process, begin by identifying the key processes (value streams) in your organization. Key processes are those that support core "products." In health care, a core product might be an office visit, or an inpatient stay, or a visit to the emergency department.

Traditional culture	Lean culture
Function silos	Interdisciplinary teams
Managers direct	Managers teach/enable
Benchmark to justify not improving: "just as good"	Seek the ultimate performance, the absence of waste
Blame people	Root cause analysis
Rewards: individual	Rewards: group sharing
Supplier is enemy	Supplier is ally
Guard information	Share information
Volume lowers cost	Removing waste lowers cost
Internal focus	Customer focus
Expert driven	Process driven

Figure E.3   Traditional culture vs. lean culture.
Source: A.P. Byrne, O.J. Fiume

For each of those core products, identify key processes, both primary and internal, that support them. Identify the person responsible for thinking about each process as a whole, how it works, and how to make it better. In most organizations, there is no one performing that role. Leaders should appoint someone who is widely respected within the organization to "own" each process in its entirety. This is not a full-time job, should not require reorganization, and needn't involve a supervisory role over those who work within the process. It does require attention to relentless pursuit of driving waste out of the process.

Lean experts note that the only sustainable process is one that participants believe in. The best way to create belief in a process is for participants to be able to see it in its entirety and to understand its logic. The best way to create vision and understanding is to directly involve participants in improving the process.

This is most often done by bringing together key participants from a chosen process in a *kaizen* event, an intensive four- or five-day session focused solely on analyzing current processes and implementing changes. (*Kaizen* means continuous, incremental improvement of an activity to create more value with less *muda*.) Large lean organizations typically conduct hundreds of *kaizen* events every year; employees know they are expected to participate, either directly on the team or testing and continuing the daily work while others participate. Some companies develop compensation mechanisms tied to *kaizen* events, or use a productivity-based compensation system so that participants feel a measure of personal investment.

For each key process identified, a *kaizen* team begins by mapping the process as it actually operates (not how it is supposed to operate), specifying value from the standpoint of the customer (external or internal), as well as waste in steps or between steps. Physically walking through the process steps—following the route of a referral form or insurance claim, for example—can be very illuminating. An example of a value stream map—in this example, for processing an insurance claim—is shown in Figure E.4. The map depicts the current process containing nine steps (as indicated in the lower left corner), with the actual required work time and elapsed process time indicated below each step in the process. Note in the lower right corner that, because of excessive delays between steps, the 19 minutes of actual work required to complete the process takes place over a 28-day period.

Next, the group envisions and maps the future state (typically within the next 12 months) by asking how the process should be changed to move toward perfection. This is known as a "future state value stream map." Figure E.5 shows a future state value stream map for the same process mapped in Figure E.4, now with only five steps in the process. Note that in the ideal future state most of the wasted time between steps is eliminated, allowing workers to complete the same 19 minutes of work in 8.3 hours instead of 28 days.

The details of these sample maps are less important than the ideas they represent. The format of a value stream map can vary according to the mapmakers' preferences. The important thing about a value stream map is that it is explicit about the flow and value of the process.

Using the future state value stream map, the group reorganizes staff if necessary to match the requirements of the process. Notice that most processes flow horizontally, while most organizations are organized vertically. This is a fundamental challenge, because the process must flow across organizational impediments and boundaries. A patient's journey from a diagnostic center to a treatment facility would be an example of this.

Like other quality improvement initiatives, implementing and sustaining the future state of a process involves Plan-Do-Study-Act

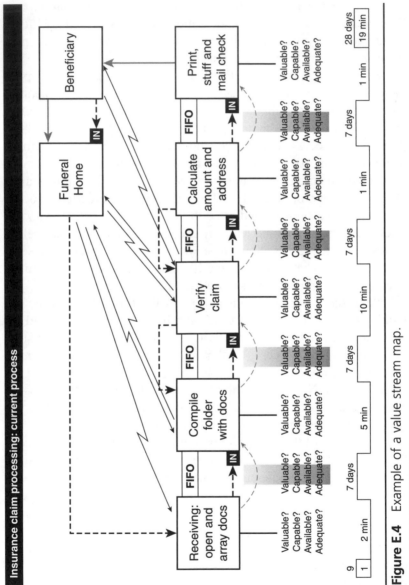

Figure E.4 Example of a value stream map.

Source: Lean Enterprise Institute

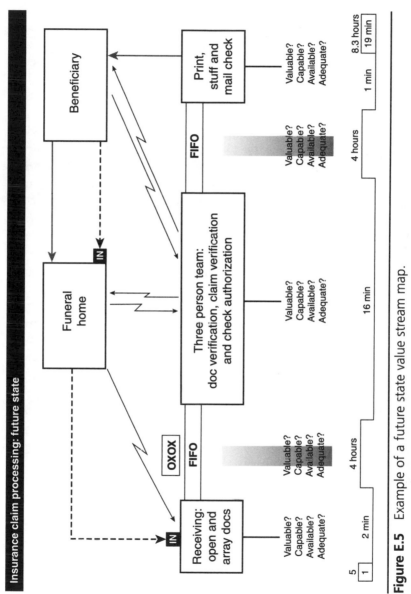

Figure E.5 Example of a future state value stream map.

Source: Lean Enterprise Institute

(PDSA) cycles in which small tests of change are carried out, the results assessed and analyzed, adjustments made, and successes spread. In trying to create a perfect process, teams should design small tests of change ("Plan"); implement the tests on a small scale ("Do"); measure the performance compared with the current state and reflect on how it could be better ("Study"); introduce the necessary changes to adjust the process ("Act"); and determine whether the adjusted process is stable and sustainable.

Continuous measurement of processes is important, as is the choice of measures, because what gets measured influences behavior. People may have an incentive to do the wrong thing if it will improve the metric. For example, a measure that focuses on the purchase price of an item might create the incentive for a purchasing manager to buy large quantities at a discount. But whether it's carburetors or catheters, excess inventory and carrying costs, along with the possibility that technical advances might render the items obsolete, create waste. "Just-in-Time" inventory is an important lean principle.

A good performance measurement system for lean processes is simple and does not include too many metrics. It supports the strategy to implement lean; motivates the desired behavior; is not overly focused on financial metrics; measures the process not the people; does not include ratios, which most people find confusing; is timely (hourly, daily, weekly) so that corrective action can be taken when the process is not going well; and uses visual displays so that people can see trends over time.

There are many additional aspects to lean thinking, more than can be covered in this paper. Readers interested in delving deeper into lean thinking are encouraged to see the list of additional resources at the end of this paper.

APPLYING LEAN THINKING TO HEALTH CARE

Virginia Mason Medical Center

Seattle's Virginia Mason Medical Center is an integrated health care system that includes a 336-bed hospital, nine locations, 400 physicians and 5,000 employees. In 2000, following a period of economic stress and a general malaise in the organizational culture, the Board of

Directors issued a broad mandate for change. Under new leadership, Virginia Mason developed a new strategic plan that called for, among other things, a sharper business focus and more accountability.

The Virginia Mason Strategic Plan is more than just words. It is mapped out in graphic form as a triangle divided into sections like the food pyramid, with the primary customer—the patient—at the top, supported equally by four "pillars": people (recruiting and retaining the best staff), quality (a focus on achieving best outcomes), service (to internal and external "customers"), and innovation (supported by the culture). The goal at Virginia Mason is to design the system and its processes around the patients' needs rather than around the needs of providers and staff. The reality is that, in lean companies, this focus on the customer also supports the staff.

The organization's vision is to be the quality leader in health care. The method that leadership chose to pursue that vision is the

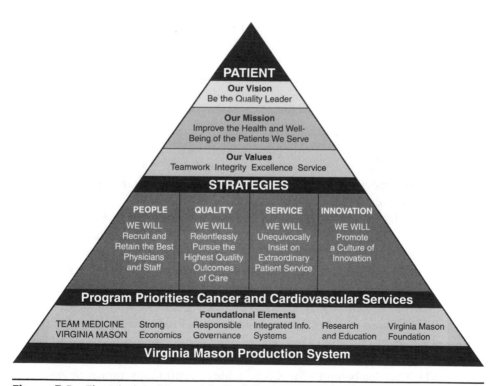

Figure E.6   The Virginia Mason Medical Center strategic plan.
Source: Virginia Mason Medical Center

Virginia Mason Production System (VMPS), modeled on the Toyota Production System. The VMPS forms the foundation for the organization's strategic plan (see Figure E.6).

Creating this strategic plan, with its clear and unequivocal focus on the patient, was the first step in changing the culture at Virginia Mason. When it was introduced in late 2001 and to this date, leaders referred to it in every presentation, relating all work to the strategic plan. Graphic images of the plan were posted in visible places throughout the organization.

In a lean environment, roles and expectations are explicit. So Virginia Mason leaders sought to clarify expectations, responsibilities, and accountabilities. In the spirit of transparency, feedback, and trust that underlies both the Toyota Production System and the Virginia Mason Production System, Virginia Mason leaders created "compacts" for leaders, for the Board of Directors, and for physicians, spelling out expectations and responsibilities for each, as well as what they can expect from the organization. This is another way that Virginia Mason laid the cultural foundation for lean.

The Virginia Mason Production System

To get all the senior leaders "on the same page" and help them immerse themselves in lean principles, in 2002 Virginia Mason sent all its senior executives to Japan to "see with their own eyes" how lean management really works. Working on the production line in the Hitachi Air Conditioning plant, executive leaders recorded workflow, measured cycle times, and documented process flow. According to senior leaders, they learned that health care has many steps and concepts in common with the production of goods.

Like health care, Japanese manufacturing processes involve concepts of quality, safety, customer satisfaction, staff satisfaction, and cost-effectiveness. The completion of the product—or the service—involves thousands of processes, many of them very complex. As in health care, the stakes are high: A product failure can cause fatalities.

Senior leaders developed the Virginia Mason Production System (VMPS), based on the principles of the Toyota Production System, following that first trip to Japan (there have been many trips since that first visit including managers, physicians, nurses and front-line staff). The idea behind VMPS is to achieve continuous improvement by adding value without adding money, people, large machines, space or inventory, all toward a single overarching goal—no waste.

VMPS has six areas of focus:

1. "Patient First" as the driver for all processes

2. The creation of an environment in which people feel safe and free to engage in improvement—including the adoption of a "No-Layoff Policy"

3. Implementation of a company-wide defect alert system called "The Patient Safety Alert System"

4. Encouragement of innovation and "trystorming" (beyond brainstorming, trystorming involves quickly trying new ideas or models of new ideas)

5. Creating a prosperous economic organization primarily by eliminating waste

6. Accountable leadership

Two details on this list bear further explanation. The No-Layoff Policy is critical to the success of implementing lean management. People will more fully commit and engage in improvement work if they are not worried about improving themselves out of a job. Attrition, typically steady in health care, will enable most organizations to reassign staff to other necessary work. A culture shift is important here as well: Staff, especially in health care, do not typically view themselves as working for the organization, but for their individual department and/or care team. In lean thinking, the patient/customer drives all processes, and staff/providers must come to understand that they work for the patient. This means they may be reassigned depending on the needs of the patients.

Secondly, the defect alert system is a fundamental element of the TPS, known as "stopping the line." Every worker in the Toyota plant has the power and the obligation to stop the assembly line when a defect or error is identified or even suspected. Workers pull a cord, a light goes on, music plays as a signal for supervisors to come and help, and the entire assembly line either slows or stops (depending on the degree of the defect resolution time) while line workers and supervisors assess and fix the problem, often preventing an error from becoming embedded in the final product. This typically happens many times a day.

The theory behind stopping the line is that mistakes are inevitable, but reversible. Defects are mistakes that were not fixed at the source, passed on to another process, or not detected soon enough and are now relatively permanent. If you fix mistakes early enough in the process, your product will have zero defects. Mistakes are least harmful and easiest to fix the closer you get to the time and place they arise. The reverse is also true.

At Virginia Mason, the Patient Safety Alert System is part of a culture in which anyone can, and indeed must, "stop the line," or stop the care process if they feel something is not right. The person who activates the alert calls the patient safety department (or submits the alert via the website) and an administrator or other relevant manager and the appropriate process stakeholders come immediately to assess the situation and conduct a root cause analysis.

In 2002 there were an average of three alerts per month at Virginia Mason; by the end of 2004 that number had risen to 17. The alerts predominately identify systems issues, medication errors, and problems with equipment and/or facilities.

An Example of a Patient Safety Alert at Virginia Mason Hospital

A Virginia Mason staff nurse noticed that a new patient had a pink wristband. A pink wristband signifies "No Code 4," meaning all resuscitation is withheld. The nurse felt this was odd because the patient had a new diagnosis of operable lung cancer, so she asked the patient what the wristband meant. The patient indicated it signified his allergy to certain medications.

The nurse replaced the wristband with the correct one—an orange one that signifies drug allergies—and reported the incident to her manager who called a Patient Safety Alert. That same day a new procedure was developed to print "Allergy Alert" on the orange wristbands.

Leadership accountability is a key component in the Patient Safety Alert System. In this instance, the Chief Nursing Officer and the Vice President of Information Systems facilitated the hospital-wide change in the wristband printing process by the following morning. When leadership goes to the *gemba,* or shop floor, changes can happen quickly.

More about the VMPS Structure and Functional Elements

The VMPS is an integrated system of processes and approaches that tie together, and must be thought of in an integrated way. A major component of the system is value stream mapping. Nearly every area in the medical center has a high-level value stream map and a detailed process flow diagram.

Kaizen events, or Rapid Process Improvement Workshops at Virginia Mason, are held weekly, bringing people together to use the tools of lean to achieve immediate results in the elimination of waste.

Other tools of VMPS include 5–S and 3–P, shorthand for organizing frameworks. 5–S (sort, simplify, standardize, sweep and self-discipline) is a method for organizing work areas to maximize smooth and efficient flow of activities and reduce wasted time and effort. 3–P (production, preparation, process) focuses on the design of new processes or workspaces.

A Sobering Reminder

In addition to the financial and efficiency gains cited earlier, the lean culture has also advanced clinical improvements at Virginia Mason. For example, because lean promotes the consistent and reliable use of standardized processes, the groundwork was laid for introduction of the "ventilator bundle," a set of specific steps proven to reduce the incidence of ventilator-associated pneumonia (VAP). In 2002, Virginia Mason had 34 cases of VAP, at an estimated cost of $500,000. In 2004, after implementing the ventilator bundle, Virginia Mason had only four cases of VAP, at an estimated cost of $60,000.

Even with these successes, leaders there say that the work of implementing lean thinking throughout the organization remains challenging, requiring considerable focus and commitment, and that despite steady progress, they are still on the journey to lean, defect-free care. This was made painfully clear in November 2004 when a Virginia Mason patient died as a result of a medical error.

Senior management, then in the process of setting its executive leadership goals for the coming year, used the tragedy as a guide in its work and reduced the proposed five executive leadership goals to just one: Ensure the Safety of Our Patients. Virginia Mason leaders believe that the Virginia Mason Production System is the means by which they can achieve this goal.

ThedaCare, Inc.

ThedaCare, Inc., is a health delivery system with three hospitals, 27 physician clinics, and a 300,000-member health plan, based in northeast Wisconsin. Nationally recognized for its quality performance results, ThedaCare is also among the nation's "most wired," or computer-savvy, health care institutions. With 5,000 employees, it is northeast Wisconsin's second largest employer.

Though some of the details differ, the "lean story" at ThedaCare is very similar to Virginia Mason's. While it is helpful to see the principles in use, it is not necessary to visit a Japanese company to gain a clear understanding of lean thinking; manufacturing companies in the US are using lean principles as well. ThedaCare leaders consulted with a nearby Wisconsin-based business, Ariens Outdoor Power Equipment Company, that has very successfully employed lean management for several years.

ThedaCare leaders set ambitious and specific goals to kindle a culture change: Improve quality to "world-class" levels (95th percentile or greater); become the health care employer of choice, making the *Fortune 100* list of best employers; and lower costs in order to lower the price paid for services, gaining $10 million a year through cost savings and increased productivity. The patient is at the center of these goals.

ThedaCare represents the goals graphically to help all staff visualize them (Figure E.7).

The culture ThedaCare leaders and staff are working to create is one in which constant improvement is seen as a never-ending jour-

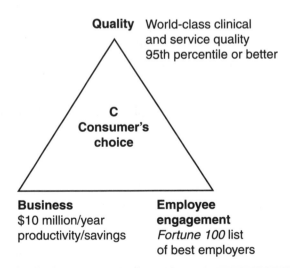

Figure E.7   ThedaCare's lean goals and metrics.
Source: ThedaCare, Inc.

ney, relying on the organization's most important attribute: the brain-power of its staff.

ThedaCare leaders recognize that a great deal of waste is the result of time the staff spend "putting out fires," and that designing processes that work better reduces waste and enables staff to better meet the needs of patients. Like Virginia Mason, ThedaCare engages staff in intensive process improvement efforts, which they call Event Weeks. Participation in at least one Event Week is mandatory for all staff members (staff can choose from six different Event Week topics each week).

The groups that come together for Event Weeks use the ThedaCare Improvement System, which includes three tenets for change, as a framework for their work. These tenets are:

1. Respect for people

2. Teaching through experience

3. Focus on world-class performance

The details of these tenets are spelled out so that leaders and staff can use them in their process improvement work. For example, Figure E.8 shows how the organization defines the first tenet.

Teaching through experience is important because people learn best when they are directly involved. The rapid results of the work— "What gets designed on Wednesday is implemented on Friday," says one ThedaCare leader—demonstrates for participants the power of their work and helps to build momentum.

What it is:	What it isn't:
Error-free practice	Long wait times
Timely service	Creating/doing non-value-added work
No waste	Wasted time
No-layoff philosophy	Wasted materials
Professionals who work together to improve performance	People focused on tasks rather than patient outcomes

Figure E.8 ThedaCare's first tenet for change: respect for people.
Source: ThedaCare, Inc.

The three goals of the ThedaCare Improvement System are:

1. Improved staff morale

2. Improved quality (reduction of defects)

3. Improved productivity

Every Event Week must focus specifically on these three goals.

ThedaCare leaders have acknowledged to staff that the new culture of lean will feel counter-intuitive for a while, with its emphasis on reducing waste and non-value-added work, as opposed to adding technology, buildings, or manpower. Lean also has a penchant for redeploying the best employees when productivity improves, not the poor or marginal performers; moving an accomplished lean thinker to a new department is an effective way to spread change.

The new culture requires new behaviors, including the use of smaller, "right-sized" groups of workers or technologies in "cells" rather than large, cumbersome processes; strong, sometimes directive leadership, augmenting more traditional team approaches; and less batching of work in favor of "right now" real-time action.

The new culture of lean also means that some roles change. For example, managers become teachers, mentors, and facilitators rather than simply directors or controllers.

Results at ThedaCare

On a monthly basis, ThedaCare tracks a range of outcomes related to lean management, including number of Event Weeks, number of employees who have participated in at least one Event Week, significant quality improvements, and financial measures.

With about six rapid improvement Event Week topics every week, by the end of 2004 ThedaCare had involved more than 600 employees directly in learning about lean thinking.

Examples of results at ThedaCare include the following:

- $3.3 million in savings in 2004

- Saved $154,000 in the Catheterization Lab supply procurement processes

- In 2004, reduced accounts receivable from 56 to 44 days equating to about $12 million in cash flow

- Redeployed staff in several areas saving the equivalent of 33 FTEs

- Improved ThedaCare Physicians phone triage times by 35 percent, reducing hold time from 89 to 58 seconds

- Reduced ThedaCare Physicians phone triage abandonment rates by 48 percent (from 11.6 percent to 6.0 percent)

- Reduced by 50 percent the time it takes to complete clinical paperwork on admission

- Appleton Medical Center Med/Surg decreased medication distribution time from 15 minute/ medication pass (the amount of time it takes to pass one medication to one patient) to 8 min/ medication pass impacting 4.1 FTEs of staff time.

CONCLUSION

Lean management is not a new concept, but it is relatively new to health care. While skeptics are right when they say, "Patients are not cars," medical care is, in fact, delivered in extraordinarily complex organizations, with thousands of interacting processes, much like the manufacturing industry. Many aspects of the Toyota Production System and other lean tools therefore can and do apply to the processes of delivering care.

Courageous, forward-thinking health care organizations such as Virginia Mason and ThedaCare, along with others, are leading the way by demonstrating that lean management can reduce waste in health care with results comparable to other industries. Leaders of these organizations emphasize the importance of creating an organizational culture that is ready and willing to accept lean thinking. Without a receptive culture the principles of lean will fail.

The Institute for Healthcare Improvement believes that many management and operations tools in other industries can be applied successfully to health care. Lean principles hold the promise of reducing or eliminating wasted time, money, and energy in health care, creating a system that is efficient, effective, and truly responsive to the needs of patients—the "customers" at the heart of it all.

White Papers in IHI's Innovation Series

① Move Your Dot™: Measuring, Evaluating, and Reducing Hospital Mortality Rates

② Optimizing Patient Flow: Moving Patients Smoothly Through Acute Care Settings

③ The Breakthrough Series: IHI's Collaborative Model for Achieving Breakthrough Improvement

④ Improving the Reliability of Health Care

⑤ Transforming Care at the Bedside

⑥ Seven Leadership Leverage Points for Organization-Level Improvement in Health Care

❼ Going Lean in Health Care

All white papers in IHI's Innovation Series are available online—and can be downloaded at no charge—at www.ihi.org in the Products section.

We have developed IHI's Innovation Series white papers to further our mission of improving the quality and value of health care. The ideas and findings in these white papers represent innovative work by organizations affiliated with IHI. Our white papers are designed to share with readers the problems IHI is working to address; the ideas, changes, and methods we are developing and testing to help organizations make breakthrough improvements; and early results where they exist.

For reprint requests, please contact:

Institute for Healthcare Improvement, 20 University Road, 7th Floor, Cambridge, MA 02138

Telephone 617-301-4800, or visit our website at www.ihi.org

INSITUTE FOR HEALTHCARE IMPROVEMENT

Appendix F

Creating Lean Healthcare

By George Alukal and Robert Chalice

Within the last 10 years or so, a new term—lean—has entered the healthcare vocabulary. Decision makers working as senior leaders, especially in executive management, nursing, quality, human resources, and operations, have been hearing a lot about lean recently in a context other than dieting.

Lean originated as a manufacturing philosophy that shortens the lead time between a customer order and the shipment of the products or parts (or the provision of requested services) through the elimination of all forms of waste. Lean is now being steadily applied to healthcare. Lean helps reduce costs, process times and unnecessary, non-value-added activities, resulting in more competitive, agile, and responsive healthcare.

The National Institute of Standards and Technology Manufacturing Extension Partnership (NIST/MEP), a part of the U.S. Department of Commerce, says lean is a systematic approach to identifying and eliminating waste (nonvalue-added activities) through continuous improvement by flowing the service or product when the patient needs it (called "pull") in pursuit of perfection.

Lean focuses on value-added expenditure of resources from the patients' viewpoint. Another description would be to give patients:

- What they want
- When they want it
- Where they want it

- At a competitive price

- In the quantities and varieties they want

- Always of expected quality

Many of the concepts in total quality management (TQM) and team-based continuous improvement are also common to the implementation of lean strategies.

WHY THE EMPHASIS ON LEAN NOW?

The reasons lean is a particularly important winning strategy in healthcare today include the following:

- The need to reduce healthcare cost and improve quality and on-time processes.

- Fast-paced technological changes

- Ever-increasing patient/customer expectations

- The need to standardize processes to consistently get expected high-quality results

IN 50 WORDS OR LESS

- Today's focus on quality and cost effective healthcare has led to renewed interest in lean.

- Lean's elimination of waste and variation makes healthcare organizations more competitive, agile and responsive to patients.

- Executive leadership, planning and implementation management are keys to successfully implementing lean.

To compete successfully in today's healthcare market, you need to be at least as good as any of your competitors, if not better. This is true not only regarding quality, but also for costs and access, processing, and other cycle times.

Lean emphasizes such things as teamwork, continuous training and learning, producing to demand (pull), personalization, batch size reduction, cellular flow, quick changeover and total productive maintenance. Not surprisingly, lean implementation uses both incremental and breakthrough improvement approaches.

The "Wastes" of Lean

Waste of resources has direct impact on cost, quality and delivery. Excess inventory, unnecessary movement, untapped human potential, unplanned downtime and suboptimal changeover time are all symptoms of waste. Conversely, the elimination of wastes results in higher customer satisfaction, profitability, throughput, and efficiency.

Eight types of waste (called *muda* in Japanese) are associated with lean:

1. **Overproduction:** doing more, earlier or faster than required by the next process.

2. **Inventory waste:** any supply in excess of short term need.

3. **Defects:** requiring inspection or rework.

4. **Overprocessing:** extra effort that adds no value to the service (or product) from the patient's point of view.

5. **Waiting:** idle time waiting for such things as staff, supplies, equipment, tests, or information.

6. **People:** not fully using people's mental and creative skills and experience.

7. **Motion:** any movement of people, or equipment that does not add value to the service or produce.

8. **Transportation waste:** transporting patients or supplies or staff around the facility more than needed.

Cutting out these eight types of waste is the major objective of lean implementation. The continuous reduction or elimination of them results in surprisingly large reductions in costs and cycle times. A root cause analysis of each of the eight wastes allows you to come up with the appropriate lean tool to tackle the causes identified.

Table F.1 Causes of variation and waste.

- Poor layout
- Long setup time
- Poor workplace organization
- Poor equipment maintenance
- Inadequate training
- Use of improper methods
- Statistically incapable processes
- Not following standardized, documented procedures
- Instructions or information unclear
- Poor planning
- Supplier quality problems
- Inaccurate tests
- Poor work environment (for example, light, heat, humidity, cleanliness and clutter)

If, for instance, long appointment lead times and missed schedules are major problems, identifying the underlying reasons might lead you to focus on such things as setup times, equipment downtime, absenteeism, missed supplier shipments, quality problems, or excess inventory.

Many examples of waste may be associated with variations in processes. Statistical tools, including Six Sigma's DMAIC (define, measure, analyze, improve, control) methodology might be appropriate to attack such wastes. Table 1 provides a look at other examples of root causes of variation and waste.

Lean and Six Sigma, thus, are not mutually exclusive—rather they are complementary. Some firms use an appropriate combination of lean, Six Sigma, theory of constraints and TQM in their constant striving for continuous improvement and competitive advantage.

Starting the Journey

The starting point of lean initiatives could be any one of the following:

- Value stream mapping
- Lean baseline assessment

- Mass training

- The basic building blocks of lean

- A pilot project

- Change management

- Analysis of internal overall equipment effectiveness and losses

Value Stream Mapping (VSM)

VSM studies the set of specific actions required to satisfy patient/customer needs, concentrating on physical transformations and information management.

The outputs of VSM are a current state map, future state map and implementation plan for getting from the current to the future state. Using VSM, you can drastically bring the total lead time closer and closer to the actual value added processing time by attacking the identified bottlenecks and constraints.

The implementation plan serves as the guide. Bottlenecks addressed could include long setup times, unreliable equipment, unacceptable first pass results, or high work or process inventories.

Lean Baseline Assessment

Using interviews, informal flowcharting, process observations and analysis of reliable data, an "as is" situational report can be generated from which the lean improvement plan flows, based on the identified gaps.

Mass Training

After training in lean is provided to a critical mass of employees in teach-do cycles, lean should be immediately implemented.

The Basic Building Blocks of Lean

These include 5S (see Figure F.1), visual controls, streamlined layout, point of use storage and standardized work. You then build on the implementation building blocks with higher level tools and techniques, finally achieving continuous patient flow based on patient needs (pull).

A Pilot Project

Choose a bottleneck or constraint area for breakthrough lean improvement using a *Kaizen* Blitz approach for breakthrough improvements. *Kaizen Blitz* intensely focuses improvement efforts on a particular process or work area over a short period, such as one week. Then, using the lessons learned, migrate lean implementation to other areas.

Change Management

Align the healthcare organization's strategies and employee goals; then change the culture from the traditional processes to lean pull. This should eventually result in a philosophical change in how daily work life is viewed.

Analysis of Internal Overall Equipment Effectiveness and Losses

A Pareto chart of these losses will identify the biggest opportunities and indicate where to start the lean journey.

Building Blocks

The tools and techniques used to introduce, sustain and improve a lean system are sometimes referred to as the lean building blocks. See Figure F.1.

A lean healthcare facility focuses on the patient to provide true value in every process step. The foundation of the lean healthcare facility includes the key structural blocks of:

- **Respect for Employees** and promoting their development. This is a critical requirement of lean.

- **Solid executive leadership** and support.

- **Continuous Improvement Teams** and kaizen events. In the lean environment, the emphasis is on working in teams, whether improvement teams or daily work teams.

- **Empathetic Change Management**, which further strengthens respect for employees.

If any these key foundation blocks are missing, the structure will fail or at least be severely compromised.

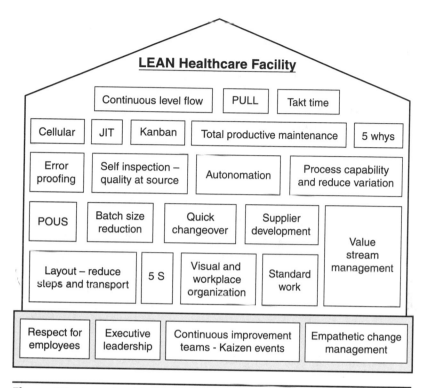

Figure F.1   Lean healthcare building blocks.

The remaining other building blocks are:

- **Workplace layout.** The workplace layout is streamlined according to optimum operational sequence to minimize steps and transport.

- **5S.** The five steps that go into this system for workplace organization and standardization all start with the letter S in Japanese (*seiri, seiton, seison, seiketsu,* and *shitsuke*). These five terms are loosely translated into English as sort, set in order, shine, standardize, and sustain.

- **Visual workplace.** All equipment, supplies, activities, and indicators are in view so everyone involved can understand the status of the system and the work processes at a glance. Equipment, instruments, and supplies are visibly stored in standard places. Work and workers remain visible so that the pace of work is clear.

- **Standard work.** Performance of a task is consistent according to prescribed methods, without waste and focused on ergonomics (human movement). Whenever possible standardized procedures and policies are posted in easy view or are easily accessible.

- **Value stream management.** A value stream is all the actions, (both value added and non-value added), that are required to deliver final value to the customer or patient. Value Stream Management focuses on delivering optimal value at lowest cost to the customer/patient within the shortest time by eliminating non-value-added steps. The goal of an organization should be to map all its key value streams and optimize them. This might be done sequentially starting with the value stream with the greatest opportunities. A manager would be assigned as responsible for the optimal functioning of each key value stream. This (horizontal) value stream manager might need to negotiate with other vertically organized managers in the organization to continuously improve a value stream.

- **Point of use storage (POUS).** Supplies, equipment, and information, work standards, procedures, and policies are stored near the staff where they are needed.

- **Batch size reduction.** The best batch size is one-piece flow. If one-piece flow is not appropriate, reduce the batch to the smallest size possible.

- **Quick changeover.** The ability to change equipment and work areas (such as ORs) usually in minutes allows for more procedures using the same resources.

- **Supplier development.** Suppliers are treated as key partners to optimize overall results. A few key suppliers that deliver top performance are relied upon and cultivated.

- **Error proofing (poka yoke).** Processes and equipment are designed to eliminate the possibility of an error from ever occurring. This prevents "accidents waiting to happen."

- **5 why's.** When an error or defect occurs, it's important to ask "Why?" five times to get to the true root cause of the problem. Otherwise one may try to correct a symptom as opposed to correcting the real cause.

- **Quality at the source.** Inspection and process control are carried out by the front line staff doing the work so they are certain the patient or product passed to the next process is of acceptable quality. Providing quality at the source eliminates the waste of re-inspection and correction.

- **Autonomation.** Machines and equipment are built with "human intelligence" and are able to detect and prevent defects. Machines stop autonomously when defects are detected, asking for help. Autonomation was pioneered by Sakichi Toyoda with the invention of automatic looms that stopped when a thread broke, allowing an operator to manage many looms without risk of producing large amounts of defective cloth. Autonomation, also known as jidoka, is a pillar of the Toyota Production System.

- **Process capability and reducing variation.** Processes are designed to produce consistently high-quality results with minimal variation or defects.

- **Cellular or flow.** The aim of one-piece flow is to physically link and arrange process steps into the most efficient combination, thus maximizing value added content while minimizing waste. Cellular flow allows one or a few cross-trained workers to perform all the functions in a well arranged work cell and to share duties.

- **JIT.** Just-in-time inventories are provided in the right amounts at the correct time and place to support ongoing processes without delay or excess supply.

- **Kanban.** Under this system of cascading processes, supply delivery instructions from downstream to upstream activities are only provided when needed, using a *kanban signaling* system. The supply request may be a kanban card or empty bin or electronic signal.

- **Total productive maintenance (TPM).** This lean equipment maintenance strategy maximizes overall equipment effectiveness. Many building blocks are interconnected and can be implemented in tandem. For example, 5S, visual controls, point of use storage, standardized work, streamlined layout, working in teams and autonomous maintenance (part of total productive maintenance) can all be components of a planned implementation effort.

- **Continuous level flow.** Production continues at an optimal steady rate. It is desirable to level demand and the needed rate of production so that level flow is maintained without overburdening employees.

- **Pull.** Downstream processes signal upstream processes to produce as needed.

- **Takt time.** This is the "heartbeat" of a steady production process. Production continues at this steady defined pace unless production is stopped to prevent the propagation of errors or defects. Takt time is also set to not overburden patients or employees.

Example

Let's look at one example in detail. If the primary reason for health-care process problems is long process changeover times, the correct tool or lean building block to use will most likely be quick changeover techniques.

Changeover time is the time between the last good output off the current run and the first good output off the next run. The traditional changeover assumption is that long runs of the same thing are necessary to offset the cost of lengthy changeovers. This is not valid if the changeover time can be made as short as possible (under 10 minutes if the quick changeover technique is applicable) and standardized at that level so there is confidence the first good output from the next run can be made in a certain period.

The changeover improvement process typically includes the following steps:

- Identify and form the changeover improvement team (such as staff, supervisors, quality specialists, setup specialists, supply handlers, maintenance technicians, and team leaders).

- Document the current changeover (videotape where possible).

- Through brainstorming, analyze the changeovers and identify ways to reduce, eliminate, consolidate or mistake-proof steps and convert from internal to external time and tasks. (Internal time is when the resource, for example, operating room is stopped, whereas external time is when the resource, for example, is running and productive with the previous case). One way to improve turnover time is to convert internal time to external time whenever possible. Thus more turnover tasks can be accomplished while the prior case is actually still in process.

- Implement improvements and monitor results.

- Streamline all aspects of setup operations.

- Standardize the improved changeover.

Besides attacking overproduction and inventory wastes, quick changeover can reduce lead time, defects and space requirements while improving productivity and flexibility and allowing more variety (customization).

Lean Enterprise

Lean healthcare implementation has slightly different challenges compared to deploying lean in manufacturing.

On the shop floor, a tangible product is being transformed. The utility of the tools and techniques for cost and cycle time reduction in processing raw materials into usable finished goods is fairly evident.

In the healthcare processes, the same Lean tools and techniques are still applicable but in a slightly modified form. Instead of hardware, you look at value adding process steps and information.

For example, you can visualize the usefulness of lean in a hospital setting, where many processes could be improved with cycle time reduction through methods such as team training, standardized work, point of use storage, visual systems and quality at the source.

Our goal is to streamline processes by purging nonvalue added steps from the time a physician (or service) order is made until the service is delivered. Bottlenecks are attacked using the plan-do-check-act model and the appropriate lean building blocks. It's of great value to identify major bottlenecks that constrain the process and then to selectively eliminate them. This allows new bottlenecks to be visible and to then be eliminated. Successive elimination of such bottlenecks results in a higher process throughput.

Eliminating Barriers

Administrators know you cannot stand still in the face of competition because your rivals are not standing pat but are improving their processes and systems to catch up with you. If you do not also improve, they will overtake you sooner or later. You lose market share, margins deteriorate, and revenue and profitability suffer. Ever increasing healthcare costs and concerns with quality also clamor for improvement.

So, if you know you need to improve, the question then becomes, why don't you?

Proper planning and implementation management are the keys to obtaining enduring success with lean deployment. Lean is not a quick fix. You are kidding yourself if you think lean implementation is easy. Success requires not only executive leadership and good change management practices, but also the integration of lean into the overall organizational strategy. The flavor of the week syndrome should be avoided. It's important to make lean operations the way the organization functions, as Toyota has done.

Complete implementation of lean might not be for everybody, so a well thought out master plan based on cost-benefit analysis is a useful preliminary step. Great benefits from lean implementation are derived by first focusing on what processes you have, the product lines that are most important to you, the environment you operate in, the competitive situation you face, and the need to use the right technique at the right time.

For lean implementation to be successful, senior managers must take an active role in many areas.

Examples include:

- Undertaking a planned approach to lean implementation, rather than single-point solutions.

- Providing needed resources.

- Appointing lean champions.

- Empowering and involving employees and emphasizing teamwork and cooperation. It's critical to recognize the value and knowledge of front line employees. Respect for employees and their experience and knowledge is key.

- Having good communication channels—both top down and bottom up.

- Managing expectations, such as fear of loss of jobs.

- Making sure everyone understands the need for change, as well as new roles as change is implemented.

- Creating an atmosphere of experimentation, a risk-taking environment and a safety net for trial and error. "Improvements" may not always work the first time as expected, but a scientific approach to improvement will.

- Offering good rewards and recognition programs, suggestion systems and gain sharing.

- Making everybody understand the competitive reasons for and benefits of lean for the organization as well as for themselves personally.

- Creating a vision of the future after the change.

- Introducing a performance measurement system based on meeting organizational goals, and rewarding them.

- Analyzing and sharing of cost vs. benefit information.

- Emphasizing everyone's accountability.

CORE CONCEPTS OF LEAN

Here are some useful concepts to keep in mind while preparing for a lean transformation:

- Creativity before capital: In lean, team brainstorming of ideas and solutions is emphasized instead of spending large sums of money on capital expenditures. People working in the process are brought together to tap into their experiences, skills and brainpower to generate a plan for waste reduction and process improvements.

- A not-so-perfect solution implemented today is better than a perfect solution that is late. Just do it now!

- Inventory is not an asset, but a cost or waste.

- Use the proven plan-do-check-act methodology for deploying improvements—both incremental and breakthrough. Plan an improvement, do it, check the results, and act to make adjustments to optimize the results. Repeat the PDCA process to continuously improve toward perfection.

- Once started, lean is a never-ending journey.

Typically, 95% of total lead time is not value added. Again, lead time is defined as the time between customer/patient request and the actual complete provision of the product or service requested. Collapsing the lead time closer to the actual processing time by squeezing out non-value-added time and tasks results in both cost and cycle time reductions. Henry Ford knew this in 1926, when he said, "One of the most noteworthy accomplishments in keeping the price of Ford products low is the gradual shortening of the production cycle. The longer an article is in the process of manufacture and the more it is moved about, the greater is its ultimate cost." Similarly, the more a patient is subjected to non-value-added activities and moved about, the greater the costs of healthcare.

In many cases, implementing pilot projects first, perhaps in a *Kaizen* Blitz mode or doing a clearly beneficial 5S project, gets immediate buy-in from skeptics. The success achieved from these quick hits can then be migrated to other areas in a planned approach. Ultimately, lean has to become the daily work habit or operating philosophy of the whole organization to be sustainable (cf. Toyota).

Starting the lean process is comparatively easy; but sustaining it over the long haul takes executive leadership, commitment, robust planning, discipline, patience, an environment that tolerates some risk or mistakes, a good reward and recognition program and peoples' receptivity to change and growth.

Many managers have found the three essential ingredients for successful lean implementation are:

- Sustained, hands-on, long-term commitment from senior management.

- Training for all employees in the lean building blocks.

- Good cultural change management during the transformation from the traditional push to the lean pull mentality.

Never-Ending Journey

Many firms have appointed and empowered lean champions for successfully implementing their lean transformation. These champions help others as mentors, trainers, group facilitators, communicators, planners, evaluators, drivers of continuous improvements and cheerleaders celebrating each success.

Champions also help in permanently capturing the gains by standardizing at the higher levels of performance as lean is implemented, so as not to slip back. Holding gains is a critical final step to prevent backsliding.

Lean will not work if it is viewed as merely a project, point solution or way of downsizing. Because lean is a never ending journey, there is always room for continuous improvement—a necessary component of any effective quality management system and the key to success in today's highly competitive and rapidly changing healthcare delivery system.

A BRIEF HISTORY OF LEAN

Most lean concepts are not new. Many were being practiced at Ford during the 1920s and are familiar to most industrial engineers.

A few years after World War II ended, Eiji Toyoda of Japan's Toyota Motor Co. visited American car manufacturers to learn from them and transplant U.S. automobile production practices to Toyota's plants.

With the eventual assistance of Toyota's Taiichi Ohno and Shigeo Shingo, Mr. Toyoda introduced and continuously refined a system of manufacturing that had a goal of reducing or eliminating nonvalue added tasks—those for which the customer is not willing to pay. The concepts and techniques that go into this system are now known as the Toyota Production System, and they were recently reintroduced and popularized in America under the umbrella of lean manufacturing.

Lean concepts are now also being applied to healthcare delivery. Lean implemented across an organization is referred to as a "lean enterprise."

George Alukal *is vice president of quality and process improvement at Chicago Manufacturing Center. He earned a master's degree in business administration from the Kellogg School of Management at Northwestern University, Evanston, IL.*

Robert Chalice *is president of the Chalice Consulting Group of Wausau, WI, specializing in lean healthcare improvements. He earned a master's degree in industrial engineering and computer science from Northwestern University, Evanston, IL, and has focused his entire career on process improvements in healthcare. He may be contacted via e-mail at authors@asq.org.*

Appendix G

Fixing Healthcare From the Inside, Today

How can health care professionals ensure that the quality of their service matches their knowledge and aspirations? As a number of hospitals and clinics have discovered, learning how to improve the work you do while you actually do it can deliver extraordinary savings in lives and dollars.

by Steven J. Spear
Steven J. Spear is a senior fellow at the Institute for Healthcare Improvement in Cambridge, Massachusetts. He is the coauthor, with H. Kent Bowen, of "Decoding the DNA of the Toyota Production System" (HBR September–October 1999), and he is the author of "Learning to Lead at Toyota" (HBR May 2004).

Last year on Christmas day, a 32-year-old Belgian woman celebrated the birth of a healthy daughter. Nothing remarkable about that, you might say, except that seven years prior, this same woman had been diagnosed with Hodgkin's lymphoma. Because doctors feared that chemotherapy would leave her infertile, they surgically removed, froze, and stored her ovaries. Once her treatment was concluded, with her cancer sufficiently in remission, they thawed the tissue and returned it to her abdomen, after which she was able to conceive and deliver.

Such medical miracles—improvements in fertility treatment, cancer cures, cardiac care, and AIDS management among them—are becoming so commonplace that we take them for granted. Yet, in the United States, the health care system often fails to deliver on the promise of the science it employs. Care is denied to many people, and what's provided can be worse than the disease. As many as 98,000 people die each year in U.S. hospitals from medical error, according to studies reviewed by the Institute of Medicine. Other studies indicate that nearly as many succumb to hospital-acquired infections.[1] The Centers for Disease Control and Prevention (CDC) estimates that for each person who dies from an error or infection, five to ten others suffer a nonfatal infection. With approximately 33.6 million hospitalizations in the United States each year, that means as many as 88 people out of every 1,000 will suffer injury or illness as a consequence of treatment, and perhaps six of them will die as a result. In other words, in the 15 to 20 minutes it might take you to read this article, five to seven patients will die owing to medical errors and infections acquired in U.S. hospitals and 85 to 113 will be hurt. Health care safety expert Lucian Leape compares the risk of entering an American hospital to that of parachuting off a building or a bridge.

How can this be in the country that leads the world in medical science? It's not that caregivers don't care. Quite the contrary: Health care professionals are typically intelligent, well-trained people who have chosen careers expressly to cure and comfort. For that reason, perhaps, many policy makers and management scholars believe that the problems with American health care are rooted in regulatory and market failures. They argue that institutions and processes mandated by law and custom are preventing demand for health care from matching efficiently to those most capable of providing it. In this view, the best treatment for what ails the U.S. health care system is strengthening market mechanisms—rewarding doctors according to patient outcomes rather than the number of patients they treat, for instance; increasing access to information about health care providers' effectiveness to employers, individuals, and insurers; expanding consumer choice.

I won't dispute the benefits of these reforms. The efficiency of health care markets may indeed be gravely compromised by poor regulation, and economic incentives should reinforce health care providers' commitment to their patients. But I fear that the exclusive pursuit of market-based solutions will cause professionals and policy makers to ignore huge opportunities for improving health care's quality, increasing its availability, and reducing its cost. What I'm talking about here are opportunities that will not require any legislation or market reconfiguration, that will need little or no capital investment in most cases, and—perhaps most important—that can be started today and realized in the near term by the nurses, doctors, administrators, and technicians who are already at work.

The scale of the potential opportunities can be seen in the results of a number of projects I've been following over the past five years at various hospitals and clinics in Boston; Pittsburgh; Appleton, Wisconsin; Salt Lake City; Seattle; and elsewhere. Consider just one example. The CDC cites estimates indicating that bloodstream infections arising from the insertion of a central line (an intravenous catheter) affect up to 250,000 patients a year in the United States, killing some 15% or more. The CDC puts the cost of additional care per infection in the tens of thousands of dollars. Yet, two dozen Pittsburgh hospitals have succeeded in cutting the incidence of central-line infections by more than 50%; some, in fact, have reduced them by more than 90%. Rolled out throughout the U.S., these improvements alone would save thousands of lives and billions of dollars.

Other hospitals have dramatically lowered the incidence of infections arising from surgery and of pneumonia associated with ventilators. Still others have improved primary care, nursing care, medication administration, and a host of other clinical and nonclinical processes. All of these improvements have a direct impact on the safety, quality, efficiency, reliability, and timeliness of health care. Were the methods these organizations employ used more broadly, the results would be extraordinary. In fact, you could read an entire issue of HBR, even several, and during that time the number of fatalities would be close to zero. (See Figure G.1)

To understand how the improvements were achieved, it is necessary to appreciate why such a gap exists between the U.S. health care system's performance and the skills and intentions of the people who work in it. The problem stems partly from the system's complexity, which creates many opportunities for ambiguity in terms of how an individual's work should be performed and how the work of many individuals should be successfully coordinated into an integrated whole. The Belgian woman's treatment, for instance, required a large number of oncologists, surgeons, obstetricians, pharmacists, and nurses both to perform well in their individual roles and to coordinate successfully with one another. Unless everyone is completely clear about the tasks that must be done, exactly who should be doing them, and just how they should be performed, the potential for error will always be high.

The problem also stems from the way health care workers react to ambiguities when they encounter them. Like people in many other industries, they tend to work around problems, meeting patients' immediate needs but not resolving the ambiguities themselves. As a

What if the improvements to medical care described in this article were adopted by every hospital in the United States? The following calculations estimate how many lives and how much money could be saved if actual rates (drawn from a number of conservative empirical studies) were cut in half—and if they were slashed by 90%.

Medical errors in U.S. hospitals		
Estimate of current annual level, nationwide	Benefit if rate were cut 50%	Benefit if rate were cut 90%
974,000 patients injured	487,000 patients avoiding injury	877,000 patients avoiding injury
44,000 to 98,000 deaths	22,000 to 49,000 lives saved	39,600 to 88,200 lives saved
$17 billion to $29 billion in costs	$8.5 billion to $14.5 billion saved	$15.3 billion to $26.1 billion saved

Figure G.1   The health care opportunity.   *Continued*

Sources: Unless otherwise noted, current figures are estimated from studies published in *To Err Is Human: Building a Safer Health System*, eds. Linda T. Kohn, Janet M. Corrigan, and Molla S. Donaldson (Institute of Medicine, 2000). Injuries from medical and medication errors are estimated from figures in Eric J. Thomas et al., "Incidence and Types of Adverse Events and Negligent Care in Utah and Colorado," *Medical Care* (Spring 2000). Central-line figures estimated from D. M. Kluger and D. G. Makl, "The Relative Risk of Intravascular Device-Related Bloodstream Infections in Adults," *Abstracts of the 39th Interscience Conference on Antimicrobial Agents and Chemotherapy* (American Society for Microbiology, 1999) cited in the CDC's August 9, 2002 weekly report of guidelines for prevention of central-line morbidity and mortality.

Preventable medication errors		
Estimate of current annual level, nationwide	**Benefit if mistakes were reduced by 50%**	**Benefit if mistakes were reduced by 90%**
785,000 patients injured	92,500 patients avoiding injury	166,500 patients avoiding injury
7,000 deaths	3,500 lives saved	6,300 lives saved
$2 billion in costs	$1 billion saved	$1.8 billion saved

Central-line infections		
Estimate of current annual level, nationwide	**Benefit if infections were reduced by 50%**	**Benefit if infections were reduced by 90%**
250,000 patients affected	125,000 patients avoiding injury	225,000 patients avoiding infection
30,000 to 62,500 deaths	15,000 to 31,250 lives saved	27,000 to 56,250 lives saved
$6.25 billion in costs	$3.13 billion saved	$5.63 billion saved

Figure G.1   *Continued*

result, people confront "the same problem, every day, for years" (as one nurse framed it for me) regularly manifested as inefficiencies and irritations—and, occasionally, as catastrophes.

But as industry leaders such as Toyota, Alcoa, Southwest Airlines, and Vanguard have demonstrated, it is possible to manage the contributions of dozens, hundreds, and even thousands of specialists in such a way that their collective effort not only is capable and reliable in the short term but also improves steadily in the longer term. These companies create and deliver far more value than their competitors, even though they serve the same customers, employ similar technologies, and use the same suppliers. Operating in vastly different industries, they have all achieved their superior positions by applying, consciously or not, a common approach to operations design and management.

As I have argued in previous articles in *Harvard Business Review,* what sets the operations of such companies apart is the way they tightly couple the process of doing work with the process of learning to do it better as it's being done. Operations are expressly designed to reveal problems as they occur. When they arise, no matter how trivial they are, they are addressed quickly. If the solution to a particular problem generates new insights, these are deployed systemically. And

---

Four basic organizational capabilities, if properly developed and nurtured, deliver the kind of operational excellence exhibited at Toyota and companies like it:

1. Work is designed as a series of ongoing experiments that immediately reveal problems. In order to drive out any ambiguity, employees in industry-leading companies spell out how work is expected to proceed in extraordinary detail, especially for highly complex and idiosyncratic processes. This increases the chance that the employees will succeed because it forces them to make their best understanding of a process explicit. If they don't succeed, spelling out what is expected increases the chance that problems will be detected earlier rather than later, since people will be surprised by the unexpected outcome. Such companies go even further by embedding tests into the work that show when what is actually happening is contrary to what was expected.

2. Problems are addressed immediately through rapid experimentation. When something does not go as expected, the problem is not worked around. Instead, it is addressed by those most affected by it. Its ramifications are contained and prevented from propagating and corrupting someone else's work. Causes are quickly investigated and countermeasures rapidly tested to prevent the problem from recurring. When those who first address a problem are flummoxed, the problem is quickly escalated up the hierarchy so that broader perspectives and additional resources are brought to its resolution.

3. Solutions are disseminated adaptively through collaborative experimentation. When an effective countermeasure is developed, its use is not limited to where it has been discovered. But that doesn't mean the countermeasure is simply rolled out as a cookie-cutter solution. Rather, people build on local insights into reducing defects, improving safety, enhancing responsiveness, and increasing efficiency by solving problems with colleagues from other disciplines and areas so that the countermeasure, and the process by which it was developed, is made explicit, can be emulated, and can be critiqued.

4. People at all levels of the organization are taught to become experimentalists. Finally, managers at companies like Toyota don't pretend that the ability to design work carefully, improve processes, and transfer knowledge about those improvements develops automatically or easily. Coaching, mentoring, training, and assisting activities constantly cascade down to ever more junior workers, thereby building exceptionally adaptive and self-renewing organizations.

Figure G.2   Delivering operational excellence.

managers constantly develop and encourage their subordinates' ability to design, improve, and deploy such improvements. (See Figure G.2)

This approach to operations can work wonders in health care, as the case studies in this article will show. We will see examples of how health care managers and professionals have designed their operations to reveal ambiguities and to couple the execution of their work with its improvement, thus breaking free of the work-around culture. We will also see how health care managers have transformed themselves from rescuers arriving with ready-made solutions into problem solvers helping colleagues learn the experimental method. I won't claim that moving to the new environment will be easy, given the complexities of the health care workplace. It will probably take some time, as well, because changes will have to be introduced gradually through pilot projects so as not to disrupt patient care. These changes will require serious commitment from health care managers and professionals at the highest levels. But the potential savings in lives alone—never mind the improved quality and increased access to health care that the dollar savings will make possible—are surely ample justification for attempting the voyage.

Let's begin by taking a closer look at what lies behind the health care tragedies we so often hear about.

AMBIGUITY AND THE WORK-AROUND CULTURE

Typically, care in a hospital is organized around functions. Issuing medication is the responsibility of a pharmacist, administering anesthesia of an anesthetist, and so on. The trouble is, that system often lacks reliable mechanisms for integrating the individual elements into the coherent whole required for safe, effective care. The result is ambiguity over exactly who is responsible for exactly what, when, and how. Eventually a breakdown occurs—the wrong drug is delivered or a patient is left unattended. Then, doctors and nurses improvise. They rush orders through for the right drugs, urge colleagues to find available room for patients, or hunt down critical test results. Unfortunately, once the immediate symptom is addressed, everyone moves on without analyzing and fixing what went wrong in the first place. Inevitably, the problem recurs, too often with fatal consequences.

Consider the story of Mrs. Grant, which comes to us from a 2002 article by David W. Bates in the *Annals of Internal Medicine.* A 68-year-old woman Bates called Mrs. Grant (all individuals' names in this article are likewise pseudonyms) had been recovering well from elective cardiac surgery when, all of a sudden, she began to suffer seizures. Her blood was drawn for testing, and she was rushed for a CT scan, which revealed no hemorrhage, mass, or other obvious cause. When she was returned to her room, caregivers saw from her blood test results that she was suffering from acute hypoglycemia, and they tried unsuccessfully to raise her blood sugar level. She quickly fell into a coma, and after seven weeks her family withdrew life support.

How could that have happened? A subsequent investigation revealed that at 6:45 on the morning of the incident, a nurse had responded to an alarm indicating that an arterial line had been blocked by a blood clot, and he had meant to flush the line with an anticoagulant, heparin. There was, however, no evidence that any heparin had been administered. What investigators did find was a used vial of insulin on the medication cart outside Mrs. Grant's room, even though she had no condition for which insulin would be needed. Investigators concluded that the nurse had administered insulin instead of heparin and that this error had killed the patient. In retrospect, the mistake was understandable. Insulin and heparin (both colorless fluids) were stored in vials of similar size and shape, with labels that were hard to read, and they were located next to each other on the cart.

Mrs. Grant's tragedy illustrates both the ambiguity that typifies many health care environments and the drawbacks of a work-around culture. The drugs were packaged, labeled, and stored the way they were because the people responsible for doing so did not understand how their decisions about such specifics might cause problems for the nurses administering the drugs. As a consequence, safety depended heavily on nursing staff vigilance. Given how fragmented and hurried nursing work is, that was asking a lot at the best of times. In Mrs. Grant's case, the timing of the mistake may have increased its likelihood, as the insulin was administered early in the morning, when the nurse might not have been fully alert, in a room that may have been dimly lit.

Mrs. Grant's nurse was certainly not the first in this hospital to have confused insulin with heparin. In fact, Bates (et al.) in a 1995 study found that for every death due to medication error there were ten injuries that weren't fatal and 100 instances where harm was averted. In other words, most of the time people make a mistake, they prevent it from harming the patient, mainly by catching themselves in time and replacing the wrong drug with the right one. Because they usually correct themselves quickly, almost reflexively, they seldom draw attention to the error. It is only after a patient dies or suffers a serious injury that the type of mistake and the factors contributing to it are subject to serious scrutiny.

Not all medical errors are the result of individuals failing in the face of challenges presented by confusing situations. Take the case, investigated by the Centers for Medicare & Medicaid Services, of a five-year-old boy who had electrical sensors surgically implanted in his brain to treat his epilepsy. Six hours after the operation, seizures began to rack the boy's entire body; anticonvulsant medication needed to be administered immediately. Yet even though several neurosurgeons, neurologists, and staff members from the medical intensive care unit (MICU) were either in the room, on call nearby, or at the end of a telephone, too little medication was administered too late. The boy suffered a heart attack 90 minutes into the seizures and died two days later.

When the investigators asked the doctors and nurses involved how the boy could have died surrounded by so many skilled professionals, they all explained that they had assumed at the time that someone else was responsible for administering the drugs. The MICU staff thought that the neurologists were in charge. The neurosurgery staff thought the MICU and neurologists were responsible. The neurologists thought the other two services had the lead. Those on the phone deferred to those at the patient's bedside.

Each of the professionals had probably been involved in hundreds of similarly ambiguous transfers of care. In those cases, however, either the patient didn't suffer an unexpected crisis or one of the parties involved stepped in and took a decisive lead. Unfortunately, the success of those sometimes heroic work-arounds concealed the ambiguity that made them necessary in the first place.

NAILING THE AMBIGUITIES

What can hospitals and clinics do to prevent such tragedies? The experience of the presurgery nursing unit at Western Pennsylvania Hospital ("West Penn") in Pittsburgh shows how organizations can make the transition from an ambiguous environment filled with work-arounds to one in which problems become immediately apparent and are dealt with as they occur.

On a typical day, the hospital's presurgical nursing unit prepared some 42 patients for scheduled surgery. On arrival, a patient registered with a unit secretary, who entered the person into the system. Then a nurse took the patient's medical history and conducted a physical examination. A critical part of this prepping job was drawing blood for testing, which provided essential information for the surgical team. Sometimes, the examining nurse drew the blood; other times, she asked a technician to do it; still other times, if something intruded on the nurse's attention, no one would do it. The result of this catch-as-catch-can procedure was that, on average, the blood work for one in six patients failed to be completed before the patient was ready to go to the operating room. This was costly in a number of ways. A delay in getting a patient to the OR meant idling OR staff, at an estimated cost of $300 per minute. It also meant delaying care—even canceling it, in some instances—for a patient who had been fasting and was anxious about the procedure.

When the unit reviewed the steps used in drawing blood, it uncovered, and then eliminated, a series of ambiguities in the process in a systematic way. First, though it was clear that blood needed to be drawn for every patient, it was often not clear to the nursing staff whether the procedure had already been done. To eliminate this confusion, the unit introduced visual indicators to identify which patients still needed the procedure and which did not. These indicators included stickers on charts and signs on the ends of beds, both of which could be deployed easily during the presurgical preparation.

But even when it was clear which patients needed blood drawn, it was not clear who should do it. The nurse? A technician? To deal with this second ambiguity, the unit designated a particular staff member, whom we'll call Mary, to be the sole person to draw blood from every patient. Mary's appointment had positive results: The number of prepped patients missing blood test results fell sharply. Nonetheless, some patients were still ready for surgery before their tests were complete.

It turned out that even if Mary knew which patients needed their blood drawn, she didn't always know soon enough to get results back in time for their surgery. To give the lab the most time to process the sample, nurses agreed that blood should be drawn as soon as a patient was registered.

This improvement also reduced, but did not eliminate, the problem. In investigating further incidents, the nursing staff found yet another degree of ambiguity. Although Mary now knew she was responsible for drawing blood once the patients were registered, she didn't always know when the registration had been completed. There was no clear signal that Mary should begin her work. To resolve this, Mary and the unit's registration secretary specified a simple, reliable, and unambiguous visual signal—a card would be placed on a rack. If no cards were on the rack, no samples needed to be taken. If one card was on the rack, a patient had been registered and was ready to have a sample taken. Two or more cards beginning to pile up on the rack was a clear sign that Mary was taking samples at a rate slower than patients were arriving.

Despite all these improvements, a few patients were still turning up for the OR without their blood work. Mary and her colleagues took another look at their process. It was clear which patients needed to have blood drawn, who was responsible for drawing the blood, and when Mary needed to draw it. What still wasn't clear was where the procedure should take place. To eliminate this final ambiguity, the unit converted a small closet into a room for drawing blood. Stored items were removed, the walls were painted, lighting was installed, supplies were stocked, and a comfortable chair was provided for patients. With this final change, the number of patients ready for the OR without blood work declined to—and stayed at—zero.

In addition to the blood-drawing initiative, Mary's unit conducted a number of similar projects to improve the reliability of work through high-speed, iterative trials. One such effort was targeted at improving patient comfort and dignity. In the past, the unit had moved patients as far along in presurgical preparation as possible to ensure that surgeons were never kept waiting. This included getting patients to change into those uncomfortable, overly revealing hospital gowns well ahead of time, which meant that they had to wait around in public for an average of 25 minutes before being given a bed.

A team in the unit spent half a day piloting a number of innovations to allow patients to delay changing until a bed was free. Team members tested out and then established signals to indicate which bed was to be available for whom, when. A changing area was created, equipped with various signs and directions designed to ensure that patients wouldn't get lost or misplace their personal effects. Before choosing the area, the team tested different rooms and screen configurations to see how well they provided privacy and made it easy to change clothes. The changes made a considerable difference. The number of patients waiting in public in their gowns at any one time fell from as many as seven to zero. Now they could wait in their street clothes with family members until beds were ready.

West Penn's improvements didn't happen because frontline workers all of a sudden started avoiding work-arounds and instead paused to construct reliable countermeasures. Much of the credit for the successes can be attributed to the problem-solving support provided by the unit's clinical coordinator, Karen, whose role was redefined in the course of the projects.

Previously, she had been the person of last resort when unit staffers couldn't construct their own work-arounds. If they couldn't get some needed paperwork, she got it; if lab tests were missing, she chased them down. Karen's new responsibilities were very different. Staffers brought all problems, including those they could work around themselves, to her attention one by one, as they occurred, rather than after the fact (if at all) in a group. Once alerted to a problem, Karen worked with whoever had raised it to investigate the causes, develop a solution, and test and validate the changes. These were not ad hoc solutions—like putting pressure on the pharmacy to rush a particular order—but rather basic changes in the design of work that were meant to entirely prevent the problem from recurring.

In the highest-performing organizations, all workers—not just those on the front line—need to be coached to learn how to reduce ambiguity systematically and how to continually improve processes through quick, iterative experiments. Thus, to help find her way into the new approach, Karen had a mentor—Alex—who worked with her several days a week. A former hospital administrator, Alex had been trained in the principles of the Toyota Production System. Alex's role was not to teach Karen how to apply to the hospital environment the widely used tools of TPS, such as andon cords or kanban cards, but rather to teach her how to develop analogous problem-solving techniques and tools that took into account the idiosyncrasies of her unit.

In the year after Karen's role was redefined, her unit identified and tackled 54 separate problems—about one a week. These varied in scope, impact, and time involved, but each followed the approach I've just described. As Figure G.3 shows, a systematic approach to

Metric	The ambiguous, work-around system	The rapid-experiment approach
Time between signing and starting registration:	Up to 12 hours	0
Time spent registering patients:	12 minutes to 1 hour	3 minutes
Time spent assembling patients' charts:	9 hours each day	2 1/4 hours
Numer of charts with unstamped pages:	35	less than 1
Nurse's time wasted as a result each day:	70 minutes	negligible
Number of gowned patients waiting on chairs in hallway:	4 to 7 at any given time	0
Time spent waiting in gowns in public:	25 minutes, average	0
Number of patients whose lab results are incomplete:	7 out of 42	0
Availability of supplies:	Some unavailable; other overstocked but past expiration	All available when, where and in the quantity required
Number of unnecessary blood bank reports issued:	10 to 11 per day	0

Figure G.3 Eliminating ambiguity and work-arounds.

eliminating problems need not take any more time than a temporary work-around.

In the moment, it may seem that when you are faced with a problem, the most effective thing to do is work around it as quickly as possible, particularly when lives are in the balance. But see how much time was saved—and how much patient care improved—when people at Western Pennsylvania Hospital stopped working around problems, and ambiguities in work processes were systematically eliminated through a series of rapid experiments facilitated by a manager.

BIG GAINS THROUGH SMALL CHANGES

The changes I've described at West Penn were individually small, but taken together they led to marked improvement in the presurgical unit's performance. That's also characteristic of change at Toyota: People don't typically go in for big, dramatic cure-alls. Instead, they break big problems into smaller, tractable pieces and generate a steady rush of iterative changes that collectively deliver spectacular results. This determination to sweat the small stuff underlies the remarkable reduction in central line–associated bloodstream (CLAB) infections achieved by the hospitals participating in the Pittsburgh Regional Healthcare Initiative (PRHI).

Used to speed the delivery of medication, central lines are intravenous catheters placed in the blood vessels leading to the heart. Infections arising from this procedure exact a terrible cost. The figures that I cited at the top of this article—250,000 patients suffering central-line infection in U.S. hospitals, with some 15% or more deaths—are only averages. The mortality rate at just one PRHI member, LifeCare Hospitals of Pittsburgh, was a staggering 40%, and the cost for each case was anywhere between $25,000 and $80,000.

The CDC has developed guidelines for the placement and maintenance of central lines. But as the PRHI professionals realized, the guidelines are generic to all hospitals and do not take into account the idiosyncratic factors of patient, place, and worker that are the root causes of individual infections. To improve their central-line processes, therefore, the PRHI hospitals decided to identify all the potential sources of central-line infection and all the local variations. As a result, the countermeasures these hospitals generated were tailored to the caseload, staffing, and special requirements of individual institutions and units. Nevertheless, the hospitals developed their countermeasures in the same way that Mary, Karen, and their colleagues did at West Penn. They responded swiftly to individual problems, testing a variety of possible solutions quickly, and those more senior took on the responsibility of enabling those more junior to succeed in the design and improvement of the work.

At Monongahela Valley Hospital, for example, a team of infection control experts documented every line placement to identify all variations and their shortcomings. They carefully monitored all line insertions, dressing changes, medication administrations through the line, and blood draws for even the minutest breaks in technique and sterility. Each time the team observed a problem with the process, it would immediately develop and test some kind of countermeasure.

Like the innovations developed at West Penn, the countermeasures these hospitals developed were all aimed at removing ambiguity and increasing specificity in the same way—specifically, at four levels of system design: system output, responsibility, connection, and method. As they did at West Penn, the changes at the PRHI hospitals were designed to make crystal clear

- who was to get what procedure (output),

- who was to do which aspect of placing and maintaining the lines (responsibility),

- exactly what signals would be used to trigger the work (connection), and

- precisely how each step in the process would be carried out (method).

For instance, several hospitals required that the central lines in all new admissions be replaced, since the histories of those lines were not known, thus simplifying output. To ensure that lines were properly placed, some units assigned responsibility only to those who had been specifically trained in each hospital's most up-to-date techniques (while expanding the size of that group through additional training).

In terms of connections, visual signals, such as stickers, were added to patients' charts and beds to trigger the removal of catheters sooner rather than later. Other such signals were used to indicate when

In their quest to eliminate central line–associated bloodstream (CLAB) infections, the hospitals in the Pittsburgh Regional Healthcare Initiative instituted a plethora of small process enhancements that together added up to dramatic improvement.

LifeCare Hospitals

Countermeasure
- Avoid femoral lines because of increased infection risk.
- Change type of disinfectant.
- Use transparent dressings to improve visibility of wound to caregivers and reduce the need for physical manipulation as part of inspection.
- Call out every hand-washing lapse.
- Have nurses ask doctors each day if catheters can be removed or placed in lower-risk sites.
- Change lines for all new admissions, since history of current line is not known.
- Report every infection to the CEO every day, and investigate each one immediately.

Result
87% reduction in CLAB infections even as the number of lines placed rose by 9.75%.

Monongahela Valley Hospital

Countermeasure
- Require that kits always be complete so that practitioners can always don full protective garb.
- Require the lab to call the moment a positive culture is identified; initiate a root cause analysis immediately.
- Avoid femoral lines.

Result
Since 2002, zero infections in medical intensive care unit (MICU), 1 in cardiac care unit (CCU). (National average is 5 infections per 1,000 line days.) Zero urinary tract infections and zero ventilator-associated pneumonias in MICU and CCU for 6 months.

UPMC Health System

Countermeasure
- Ensure hand-washing compliance.
- Improve barrier kits and use them in a consistent manner.
- Allow medical residents to place lines only with supervision until they all are formally trained.

Result
One MICU went without a CLAB infection for several months. Systemwide rate cut to 1.2 infections per 1,000 line days.

Figure G.4 Combining countermeasures has a big effect.

Continued

Allegheny General Hospital

Countermeasure
 • Investigate each infection as it's discovered.
 • Remove all femoral lines within 24 hours.
 • Prohibit rewiring of dysfunctional lines.
 • Remove all catheters for transferred patients.
 • Use biopatch dressings for lines that are expected to be in place for two weeks or more.

Result
 Infections down from 37 in 2003 to 6 in 2004; deaths down from 19 to 1 in the same period. Direct cost reduction of $1.4 million.

Figure G.4   *Continued*

---

a catheter should be moved from a place on the body known to have a high risk of infection to a lower-risk area and to otherwise clarify when lines had to be maintained or replaced. Transparent dressings were used to make it easier to tell whether a wound site was healthy or not.

As for methods, changes were made in disinfectant materials and techniques, and the kits in which line maintenance supplies came were repeatedly modified. (One alteration was to pack gloves on the top of the kit so that people would not contaminate other components in getting at the gloves.) Tests were made of various sized surgical drapes to determine which were not so small as to be ineffective or so big that they were knocked out of place when patients moved.

The results of the initiative were impressive (see Figure G.4). At Allegheny General Hospital alone, the number of patients suffering from central-line infections declined from 37 in one year to six in the following year, and associated deaths fell from 19 to one. (To see the cumulative effect, see Figure G.5)

SIMULATION AND EXPERIMENT

On any given day, Toyota employees engaged in design and production will be conducting some kind of simulation or experiment with workers and managers, repeatedly figuring out how to test ideas as quickly and inexpensively as possible. People bolt what they would otherwise weld, tape what they would otherwise bolt, and just hold in

In less than three years, using techniques adapted from the Toyota Production System, the Pittsburgh Regional Healthcare Initiative slashed the number of reported central line–associated bloodstream (CLAB) infections by more than 50%. The rate per 1,000 line days (the measure the hospitals use) plummeted from 4.2 to 1.9.

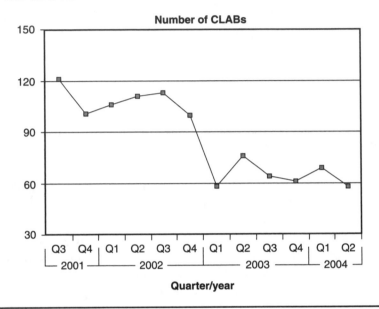

Figure G.5   Radically reducing infection

place what they would otherwise tape. The objective is to compress the time between when an idea is formulated and when it is tested.

The pharmacy at the University of Pittsburgh Medical Center (UPMC) South Side hospital used this approach in identifying and solving problems with its medication delivery process. The pharmacy was supposed to make timely deliveries of medication throughout the hospital so that nurses could administer drugs to their patients according to the appropriate schedule. But when nurses went to get the medications, they often found that what they needed was missing. This triggered work-arounds. Nurses would interrupt their work to call the pharmacy, requiring pharmacy staff to stop what they were doing to track down orders: Had they been received? Had they been entered? Had they been prepared? Had they been delivered? Where was the missing medication? How quickly could it be rushed to the person needing it? Tracking down a missing medication, with all the attendant interruptions, could consume hours of nurse, pharmacist, and technician time.

The problem, the pharmacy realized, was that medication administration was done in batches. Physicians would make rounds early in the morning—before office hours or surgery—and follow up throughout the day. As patients' conditions changed, doctors would write further orders for medication, which would be collected and delivered periodically to the pharmacy. There, pharmacists would enter the orders into the computer system, their expertise allowing them to identify potential problems with dosage, interactions, allergies, and the like. Orders would accumulate in the computer system throughout the day and then be printed out for all patients in the late afternoon. The next day, the pharmacy staff would begin filling these orders, assembling the proper mix and volume for each patient. This work would be completed in the early afternoon, at which point, a delivery technician would bring the completed orders to the nursing units. In view of the 12 to 24 hours that elapsed between the writing and the filling of an order, it was quite likely that medication needs would change, triggering work-arounds to get patients the right medicines, as well as a lot of unnecessary work restocking the old orders and making sure that patients were not billed for drugs they no longer needed.

The temptation in these situations is to brainstorm your way to an answer, with everyone proposing solutions drawn from his or her personal experience. But this was not the approach chosen here. As a first step in determining how to fix the medication preparation process, the pharmacy staff sat down as a group to determine what demands the nursing units were actually placing on the pharmacy. They counted out the previous day's orders, divided that by the number of hours the pharmacy operated, and concluded that if the pharmacy were operating at the pace at which medication was being consumed, it would have to produce and deliver one order every three minutes. This gave them a concrete goal—instead of asking what changes they needed to make the process "better," they asked what specifics prevented them from performing perfectly.

To answer that question, they set up a simulation. One pharmacist and one technician were lined up in the pharmacy, and every three minutes they were handed one order, which they tried to fill. This being an experiment, the staff used the previous day's orders, not that day's, and they delivered the medication into a cardboard box rather than having a delivery technician bring the medication all the way to the nursing unit. A stopwatch was started, a colleague handed the pair the first order, and they filled it. Three minutes later, the pharmacist and technician were handed a second order, which they filled. They were handed a third order, but before they could complete the work of finding the medication in inventory, taking out the right sized dose, labeling it, checking it, and bagging it, the three-minute interval had elapsed, and they were handed the fourth order.

At this point, they halted the experiment and asked themselves: "Why couldn't we fill the third order?" This question was critical, and semantics mattered. Asking "Why *didn't* you do your work?" elicits a very different response, typically a defensive explanation about how hardworking someone is, how he isn't trying to fail, and so on. Asking why one *couldn't* fill the order elicits a specific impediment, such as some ingredient being stored too far away or someone's handwriting being too hard to read.

In this case, the pair realized that they couldn't fill the order because the medication they were seeking couldn't be found, and by the time they were done searching for it, their time was up. That very specific reason was recorded—"medicine X was in an uncertain location"—and the experiment resumed. A new order was handed to the team, and it was filled. Three minutes passed. Another order, another successful delivery to the cardboard box. Three more minutes. Another order—and another problem. When one of them tried to take a label off the printer, it jammed, delaying the process and preventing the team from keeping pace—another specific problem to be solved. The process of trying to fill one order every three minutes continued throughout the morning, and by the lunch break the experimenters had dozens of very specific answers to why the pharmacy couldn't fill each order in time.

Some of the problems were easy to fix, such as storing drugs according to how frequently they were used rather than alphabetically. Others were more complicated, such as changing the timing at which drugs left the pharmacy, the delivery route technicians took through the hospital, and the way orders were placed with distributors. But simple or complex, the changes had a big cumulative impact. The pharmacy was ultimately never able to process and deliver each order individually, largely because the doctors writing the orders tended to do so in batches as they made their rounds, and delivery techs could not run so many individual orders to their various destinations at the same time. But the pharmacy did manage to process batches of medication once every two hours instead of once every 24 hours. As a result, the incidence of missing medications in the wards dropped 88%.

The savings in terms of pharmacy time and medication management were equally impressive. Time spent searching for medication fell by 60% and stock-outs fell by 85%—with no investment in technology. Overall medication inventory was reduced, and medication costs dropped because drugs were less likely to be lost, spoiled, or wasted. Under the old system, for instance, IV medications were delivered as much as 48 hours *before* they were actually needed. That was problematic because many IV medications had to be refrigerated or otherwise kept in a controlled fashion, taking up valuable storage space in nursing units. What's more, a patient's condition often changed before the IV was to be administered, so more than 30% of IV medications were returned to the pharmacy. Since some medications spoil quickly once mixed with a saline solution, the pharmacy staff was often obliged to throw out the returns. Under the new process, IV medications were prepared and delivered shortly before being needed, significantly reducing both waste and demands on storage in the wards.

What happened after the UPMC South Side experiment was almost more interesting than the experiment itself. When OR support staffers at UPMC Shadyside hospital learned of the improvements at South Side, they tried to apply the same tools and practices. But they soon discovered that the South Side solutions were inappropriate because of differences in the two organizations' work. So the Shadyside people visited South Side and walked through the simulation process I've just described. As they did so, they came to see that what they needed to do was master the problem-solving *process* rather than the problem-specific *solutions*. Accordingly, they set up a similar experiment at their own site, uncovered different problems, and found different solutions.

THE MODEL LINE APPROACH

When organizations first analyze their problems, they are inevitably tempted to roll out their solutions throughout the organization by installing a common set of tools and procedures broadly and quickly. But there are a couple of difficulties with that approach.

First, as Shadyside discovered, the solutions from one situation may not apply in another. Second, the most effective changes—at West Penn, South Side, and elsewhere—are small ones, generated by rapid experiments. Draw too big a group into the initial deployment, and the experiments become unwieldy, requiring too many people to change too much of their work at the same time. After all, even a small nursing unit includes several nurses in each day, evening, and night shift, as well as fill-ins for weekends, vacations, and the like and dozens of doctors who can admit patients to the unit. Finally, what sets companies like Toyota apart is not their portfolio of existing solutions but their ability to generate new ones repeatedly. One way to hone that ability is through the "model line" concept—creating, essentially, a model of the production line, a small incubator within the larger organization in which people can develop and practice the ability to design and improve work through experiments, and managers can rehearse their roles in facilitating this ongoing problem-solving and improvement process.

Shadyside used the model line approach with great success in its efforts to raise several aspects of the quality of its care. Rather than swamp the staff with a large initiative, the hospital began with a few beds within a single nursing unit and at first addressed just one of the many problems affecting nurses' ability to care for patients.

Like many hospitals, Shadyside found that its nurses spent a disproportionate amount of time nursing not the patients but the system—tracking down materials, services, and information. One consistent aggravation was with patient-controlled anesthesia (PCA) pumps. Nurses needed access keys to adjust dosages, but for security reasons the pharmacy had assigned the unit only a few keys, which were often hard to find. So, as a work-around, the nurses would go looking for the most recent user. Nurses in each shift searched for keys to the narcotics cabinet on average 23 times, wasting 49 minutes a shift and delaying pain relief to patients.

In discussing the problem, the nurses quickly realized that the limited number of keys was the issue. A nurse needing a key would check it out with the unit secretary but often fail to return it when rushing to meet another patient's needs. The solution piloted was to have a numbered key available for every nurse, which would be signed out at the beginning of the shift and signed back in only when the nurse left the unit or ended his or her shift. In this way, the pharmacy's need to control drug access was satisfied without inconveniencing the nurses. The time spent searching for keys was reduced to almost zero, and the practice was subsequently deployed throughout the hospital, saving an estimated 2,900 nurse-hours each year.

The nurses in the unit then applied their problem-solving approach to another issue: patient falls. An estimated 2% to 4% of patients fall during their hospitalization in the United States every year (which translates into 670,000 to 1.3 million individuals) and 2% to 6% of those spills (13,000 to 78,000) lead to injury. At Shadyside, the average was one fall every 12 hours. When the nurses looked into the problem, they realized that they hadn't made it clear who was at risk of falling. What's more, patient escorts were not trained in helping patients in and out of beds or on and off gurneys. That meant escorts would leave patients to find a trained nurse. Bit by bit, the unit's nurses introduced changes, in much the same way the West Penn team did. When they first arrived at the unit, patients were rated at risk or not. Escorts were taught how to safely transfer patients so that they wouldn't have to leave patients unattended. Danger areas were clearly marked (for instance, labels that said, "Don't leave me alone!" were placed by bedside toilets). Nurses and nurse assistants built into their work the regular inquiry, "Do you need to use the bathroom?" so patients wouldn't try to get out of bed on their own. Sensors were placed on beds to indicate if a patient was trying to get out of bed unassisted. And patients who needed but arrived without walkers or canes were lent the equipment they needed. After the changes were introduced, the number of falls declined dramatically—at one point, the unit went 95 days without one.

The nurses' success with PCAs and falls was not lost on the staff from the dietary department serving the same unit. The problem facing the dietitians was that they could not tell how well patients adhered to the dietary regimens appropriate for their medical conditions. Patients on restricted diets would cheat ("I can't eat this tasteless mess: Honey, can you grab me a burger, fries, and shake from the cafeteria downstairs?"). Even if patients did stick to the regimen in the hospital, they often stopped when they left, potentially compromising their recovery.

After discussing the problem-solving approach with the nurses, the dietitians realized that they could use patient meals as a way to identify precisely which patients would need further education. Rather than restrict choices, they decided to let the patients in the unit pick from the hospital's entire menu—a counterintuitive approach if your objective is to control what patients eat but not if your objective is to teach patients how to select wisely and discover when your efforts have not succeeded. Allowing patients to choose from the whole menu was coupled with counseling from dietary and nursing staff about what foods should be chosen or avoided. Menu selections were coded—with a "healthy heart" sticker, for example, to indicate low-fat options—to make it clear which choices were appropriate for the various restricted diets. Then, after patients ordered food, dietitians would compare the orders with the instructions in the patients' charts. Inappropriate picks—say, a cardiac patient ordering a high-cholesterol meal—would be treated as problems, and dietary and nursing staff would visit every problem patient before the meal was even served to provide nutritional instruction. If, after repeated counseling, patients continued to make choices contrary to recommendations, dietary and nursing staff would inform their doctors, who could modify their postdischarge medication orders appropriately, changing, for example, the type or dosage of blood pressure medication for a patient who wouldn't cut his sodium intake.

Conemaugh Health System in west central Pennsylvania used an interesting variant of the model line approach to reveal problems that spanned the boundaries of individual units and departments. To find out what was falling between the cracks, the hospital tracked the treatment of certain patients all the way from admission to discharge.

One patient had come for a cardiac catheterization following symptoms that included chest discomfort. Testing revealed no blockage, and the patient was scheduled for discharge. From the patient's perspective, this was a happy outcome, but from the hospital's perspective, the findings were sobering: The team dealing with the patient documented that fully 27 distinct and potentially dangerous problems had occurred. While none actually compromised the care given to this particular patient, team members didn't want to leave the ambiguities that caused the problems in place to be worked around again, so they worked with the pharmacy, the lab, and other departments to resolve them.

INSTITUTIONALIZING CHANGE

If one asks the question, Can the Toyota Production System be applied in health care? the quick answer is yes. The experiments I've just described all demonstrate that possibility. But to realize the full potential of TPS, senior health care leaders—hospital CEOs, presidents, chiefs of staff, vice presidents for patient care, medical directors, unit directors, and the like—will need to do more than provide support for pilot projects. They will need to embrace and embody TPS in their own work. An example from the Virginia Mason Medical Center (VMMC) illustrates what it means for managers to try to master this new approach.

VMMC is a 300-bed, Seattle-based teaching hospital with 5,400 employees and 400 physicians who admit some 16,000 patients a year and serve more than a million outpatients at ten sites. VMMC's management first became interested in TPS in 2001, after executives from local businesses described the dramatic improvements they had achieved in quality, customer satisfaction, safety, staff satisfaction, and, not least, profitability. At the time, VMMC was in sorry straits. The hospital was struggling to retain its best people, and issues of quality, safety, and morale were on everyone's mind.

VMMC started by piloting a few projects along the lines I've described in previous sections. But managers didn't really understand the potential of establishing a continuously self-improving organization until the hospital's chairman and its president, together with its professional and physician executives, went in 2002 on a two-week visit to Toyota factories, during which they all took part in an improvement project at a Toyota affiliate. Impressed by the knowledge that it was possible to establish such an organization, VMMC formally adopted TPS as a model for its management system and began to train all of its staffers in its philosophy, principles, and tools. That included a public commitment to retain all full-time employees so that people would not feel that they were expected to improve themselves out of a job.

Since then, VMMC's leadership has taken a number of steps to reduce tolerance for ambiguity and work-arounds and to make change a regular part of work. To help institutionalize a role for process experts in an organization otherwise filled with experts within disciplines, VMMC created Kaizen Promotion Offices, which support the improvement efforts of its various divisions. To emphasize the idea of quick, constant change, VMMC has conducted several hundred rapid-improvement projects. To make it easy not to work around problems, VMMC created a patient safety alert process, which allows any employee to immediately halt any process that's likely to cause harm to a patient. There's a 24/7 hotline for reporting problems, a "drop and run" commitment from leadership at the department-chief and vice-president levels to immediately respond to the reports and to exhibit a willingness to stop processes until they are fixed. To further bolster the connection between leadership and the "shop floor," department chiefs and managers conduct safety walkabouts, asking staff to alert them to specific instances in the previous few days of events that prolonged hospitalization, caused a near miss, harmed a patient, or compromised the efforts of people to do their work. Such alerts rose from three per month in 2002, the year the patient safety alert process started, to ten per month in 2003, to 17 per month in 2004. Despite the increase in the number of alerts, the average time to resolution declined from 18 days in 2002 to 13 in 2004.

This commitment to process improvement has indeed increased quality and reduced costs. In 2002, for instance, 34 patients contracted pneumonia in the hospital while on a ventilator, and five of them died. But in 2004, only four such patients became ill, and just one died. Associated costs dropped from $500,000 in 2002 to $60,000 in 2004. And the overall number of professional liability claims plummeted from 363 in 2002 to 47 in 2004. Improved efficiencies in labor, space, and equipment allowed VMMC to avoid adding a new hyperbaric chamber (saving $1 million) and avoid moving its endoscopy suites (saving another $1 million to $3 million), even as it increased the number of patients its oncology unit treated from 120 to 188.

❖   ❖   ❖

So far, no one can point to a single hospital and say, "There is the Toyota of health care." No organization has fully institutionalized to

Toyota's level the ability to design work as experiments, improve work through experiments, share the resulting knowledge through collaborative experimentation, and develop people as experimentalists. But there's reason for optimism. Companies in a host of other industries have already successfully followed in Toyota's footsteps, using common approaches to organizing for continuous learning, improvement, and innovation that transcend their business differences. And these approaches have been successful when piloted in health care.

More to the point, the health care system is populated by bright, dedicated, well-intentioned people. They have already demonstrated a capacity to experiment and learn in order to master the knowledge and skills within their disciplines. One can imagine few people better qualified to master the skills and knowledge needed to improve processes that span the boundaries of their disciplines.

Appendix H

Lean and Healthy*

A quiet revolution is beginning in Great Britain that could have profound effects on hospital management and the future of patient care. As Andrew Scotchmer discovers, the National Health Service (NHS) is taking some lean lessons from Toyota

by Andrew Scotchmer

A Japanese automobile manufacturer may not seem the most obvious mentor for cash-strapped †NHS trusts looking for guidance on efficiency improvement and quality management. Yet with debts in excess of £500 million ($935 million) that is exactly the direction they're heading.

Toyota's production system, or "lean" as it has become known in the west, needs little introduction. Beginning in the Toyota plants of the 1950s, today it is a method that has proven itself in manufacturing industries and service sectors worldwide. In a nutshell, it involves the shortening of lead time by removing all unnecessary,

---

*This article first appeared in the August 2006 issue of *Qualityworld*, the magazine for the Institute of Quality Assurance (http://www.iqa.org/publication).
†NHS—National Health Service of Great Britain. To see lean improvement examples from the NHS please go to www.institute.nhs.uk/ServiceTransformation/Lean+Thinking/

non-value adding steps and by eradicating, or at least diminishing, waste and wasteful activities. The outcome of all this waste removal is an enhanced flow of work within the production cycle. According to one of its founders, Taiichi Ohno, it is shortening the timeline from order through to payment. Any wasteful activity or process that does not add value or increases that timeline should be removed leaving only the essential value-adding processes remaining.

In their book *Lean Thinking,* Womack and Jones identify lean's five main areas: value; the value stream; flow; pull; and perfection, the ultimate goal. Each is mutually supportive of the others and together they increase efficiency and accuracy in the work place at lower costs than conventional manufacturing systems.

KEY CONCEPTS

- Muda: the Japanese term for waste. Taiichi Ohno described seven forms of waste: inventory, waiting, overproduction, unnecessary transporting, unnecessary movement, defects, and unnecessary possessing.

- Kaizen: continuous improvement of system processes through slow incremental change and review.

- Kaikaku: also termed a "kaizen blitz." Kaikaku is a rapid change to processes in order to improve the current system and receive immediate benefits. Often includes radical ideas that involve creative changes to the process. Takes place over a five-day workshop.

- Just-in-time: providing what is needed when it is needed and not before, which only produces inventory, and definitely not after.

- Kanban: a signaling device such as display boards and information cards that indicate when you are ready for more work (closely linked to just-in-time).

- Heijunka: "production leveling." Averaging out demand over a set time period. This can be a challenge in a busy and unpredictable hospital environment.

- Jidoka: a method for "building in quality." The empowerment of all staff to raise nonconformances when defects have occurred and to become involved in their solution.

What, though, does all this have to do with the NHS, an organization completely different in its structure and purpose to an industrial or manufacturing plant? Can these manufacturing methods really offer hope to struggling hospitals?

It was in the U.S. that lean methods were first used within a healthcare environment. One of the forerunners was the heavily publicized Virginia Mason hospital in Seattle. In 2001, Virginia Mason needed to quickly improve its services as debts were mounting, staff morale was plummeting, and neighbouring hospitals were beginning to steal customers.

After a coincidental meeting with Ian Black, the then lean director of Boeing, Gary Kaplin, CEO of Virginia Mason, became convinced that lean production was the solution. In 2002, Kaplin and a team of executives and managers began annual trips to Japan to study at the Shinjijutsu International Centre, one of the world leaders in the Toyota production system. On their return, staff immediately put into practice what they had learned and the benefits of implementing this new way of managing hospitals and patient care. Inventory costs were slashed by 51 percent and lead times were reduced by 708 days. Gains in productivity freed up 77 full-time equivalents (the number of full-time employees) with many being reassigned work in the newly developed lean promotion office. Defects in patient care reduced by 47 percent while kaikaku workshops saved the hospital over U.S. $12 million during the period 2002 to 2004 (see Kaikaku in Key Concepts).

One change made in just five days using the kaikaku technique concerned the delay between a doctor's referral to a specialist and the first consultation. By examining the process closely it was found that the secretaries, whose job it was to arrange these referrals, were not needed. Instead the doctor would page or text the consultant the instant he decided a specialist was required. This specialist then had to respond in 10 minutes, even if just to confirm receipt of the text. Delays in referral to treatment dropped by 68 percent as a consequence.

On another occasion, staff in the radiation oncology department began an exercise looking at and mapping out the value stream with the intention of eliminating all the waste they could find. Due to the removal of these unnecessary non-value-adding activities, which only soaked up resources, the time a patient spent in the department fell from three quarters of an hour to just 15 minutes.

Such has been the huge success at Virginia Mason that it is now a benchmark in hospital management throughout the United States. The Virginia Mason production system, or the VMPS as it has now come to be known, has even been included as a core case study for graduates on the Harvard MBA course. According to Dr Kaplin: "After you have tried it you will never go back."

THE NHS REVOLUTION

The NHS has been slower to fully embrace lean thinking but is now rapidly making up for lost time. Last January saw the first lean healthcare forum in Birmingham and a second was held in June. Chaired by author and prominent lean thinker Dan Jones, these forums have helped explain and consolidate lean knowledge.

One NHS organization that has begun the lean journey is Bolton Hospitals NHS Trust. Under the direction of CEO David Fillingham, lean has found its way into every department and management decision, reducing waste wherever it occurs and adding value to each step along the patients' care pathway. Staff too have become more motivated and focused on providing quality care to patients, with each employee responsible for analysing what they do and how they can do it better.

Lean has also been successful in decreasing the length of time inpatients stay in the hospital from an average of 34.6 days to just 23.5. The principal method for bringing about these changes involved looking at the whole supply chain's value stream as the patient traveled along his or her unique care pathway. Often, in organizations, change happens in a piecemeal fashion with separate departments initiating changes independently.

A lean approach, on the other hand, requires departments to consider from the start their positions in the supply chain and any impact their changes will make on the whole. By ensuring that all the necessary supporting services, such as health records, pathology and secretarial services, work together and come into play at just the right time, the patient, after entering the hospital and beginning the journey, does not need to be kept waiting between processes.

The patient moves or, rather, flows through the system. As one set of processes or treatment finishes another clicks into place immediately.

The Bolton Hospitals and NHS trust has also enjoyed some dramatic changes which have been made to its accident and emergency department and pathology lab, which now operates in half the space it used previously.

DOING THE KAIZEN BLITZ

As with the Virginia Mason hospital, Bolton has used the kaikaku technique for implementing rapid change. These multidisciplinary workshops aim to fix a problem in just five days with the new system up and running by the following Monday.

The way it works is quite simple. On the first Monday, a team made up of the department under review, for example radiology, and members from various departments immediately before and after in the supply chain, get together and map the current processes.

The next day, the ideal future state map is drawn up with all wastes identified and removed leaving the following days free for implementation strategies. The idea is that by Friday all the problems will have been solved and a new method of working will have been discovered and implemented ready to begin the following week.

When redesigning the blood science laboratory at Bolton, the team even invaded the hospital's car park and used cardboard cutouts of the equipment to map their ideal positions in the lab. They have managed to decrease the number of physical steps it now takes a technician to process a patient's blood sample. Fewer steps equal less walking time, which means a speedier service. Consequently, blood sample turnaround times have dropped by 90 percent.

SPREADING THE WORD

Another NHS hospital has recently shown an interest in using lean across its entire regional health economy, from the primary care suppliers at one end of the supply chain, to the local government's social services department at the other. Within its pathology department the focus has been on how specimens arrive and are sorted prior to analysis. After only two days of observation in this hospital's pathology reception area, it was concluded that the time spent processing specimens by the assistants could be reduced by 60 percent while still meeting demand.

According to biomedical scientists in the blood science lab, work cannot begin on specimens until the patient's information that accompanies the sample has been entered into the laboratory computer system by lab assistants. Sometimes the delay can be two hours between the blood being prepared for examination and the inputting. Often these highly trained and highly paid biomedical scientists can be found inputting the patients details themselves just so that they may begin work.

The newly proposed system would eradicate this problem and aid the timely investigation and reporting of blood samples to clinicians. By utilising a kanban system along with just-in-time, bloods and patients details would be processed, inputted, and ready for analysis in just 15 to 20 minutes after arrival at the laboratory.

To achieve these results it was noted how the available resources were not being used to their full potential. Blood sciences receive, on average, 1,250 specimens each day. The reception area contains three centrifuges, each holding 40 specimens. Bloods are spun in these centrifuges for 10 minutes; therefore 720 specimens could be spun in one hour. Unfortunately this solution would leave little time for any other work that needs attending to and relies on all the day's specimens arriving at once, which does not happen.

Taking a more realistic view of the situation, if each of the six assistants were allowed to concentrate on just 20 specimens at a time, half a centrifuge per assistant, patient details could easily be booked on to the computer while the blood samples were spinning. This would mean that after just 20 minutes, 120 specimens would be ready for analysis with all the necessary data in the computer. Cover is provided by the assistants for 10 hours, therefore by working only 20 minutes in each hour, demand could be met and the flow of specimens increased.

On loading the bloods onto the analysers the scientist would leave the empty test-tube rack as a visible symbol, a kanban, that more work was needed and the process would start again.

Other hospitals which have tried lean find similar successes. The Osprey program, established in 2003, involved six strategic health authorities. Its objective was to aid hospitals in applying manufacturing principles to their own care environments. The costs of running the program came to £600,000 ($1.1 million) in its first year. However, it also managed to generate a return of £9.4 million ($17.6 million) in efficiency savings.

After a kaikaku workshop and value stream mapping event, the Hereford Hospitals NHS Trust claimed that the three- to four-month waiting list for preoperative assessments was slashed to 30 minutes using lean techniques. The trauma discharge team with the same trust admitted to learning a whole new way of planning patient care.

PRINCIPLES OF LEAN

- Value: defined by the customer and produced by the supplier or manufacturer. In a healthcare setting it is what happens to aid patients along their care pathways. Processes can be defined as value adding or non-value-adding (causing delays and lengthening lead time).

- Value stream: the order of value adding processes arranged in sequential order. Value stream mapping is the first step in applying lean. The value stream helps analyze processes from the patient's point of view.

- Flow: products moving unhindered from one process to another. This could refer to specimens moving through a lab or patients "flowing" through the hospital.

- Pull: rate of work being dictated by the customer. Traditionally it was the processes behind that pushed work through the production cycle. Pull sees things from the opposite end and "pulls" production towards the customer.

- Perfection: the ultimate goal where all four principles work in total harmony, mutually supportive, internally consistent.

PATIENTS ARE NOT CARS

Critics of lean healthcare initiatives argue that people are different to cars and have different needs. Obviously this is true, but it is simply a method of working which is being adapted. Some doctors have argued that cost is secondary to health and resist the pressure to comply with what they see as a production method with no relevance to hospitals.

The chief economist at the King's Fund health think tank, John Appleby, argues that efficiency programs have often meant patients spending less time with doctors, which is, indisputably, an important part of the care process.

Though these points are valid they are also slightly off target. The systems and processes that underpin a smooth, swift patient journey do need to be addressed. For example, a doctor spending 30 minutes talking to a patient is half an hour of value added time and will be seen as such by the patient. However, if 20 minutes of that half an hour was spent looking for the patient's case notes, has the physician really given value?

Using techniques such as just-in-time to ensure that everything needed for the patient's treatment—case notes, lab results, and so forth—arrives just as it is required will improve the overall experience and quality of care. Patients will not be left to wait before moving on to the next stage of their treatment plan and will find their length of stay in hospital dramatically reduced. Doctors and nurses will find they have the time to devote to patients that currently they are unable to give due to inefficiencies within the supporting services. Lean as a manufacturing philosophy puts the customer—the patient—first.

A £500 million ($936 million) overspend may sound like a lot of money and it is but this figure pales in relation to the expected £98 billion ($183 billion) of government funds that will have been invested since coming to power by 2008. According to *The Economist,* this is in return for just a 3 percent increase in activity. Gill Morgan, CEO of the NHS confederation, remarked that any extra request for funding would fall on deaf ears until "we cut out waste in the system."

From early trials, lean certainly offers a solution. But to be truly successful, it must permeate the whole organization from the very top down. Lean is a process-based method that looks at the interactions across whole supply chains. There is little use in wards and departments attempting kaikaku or kaizen events without the full support of others positioned either below or above them in the supply chain. Neither is it feasible that lean will supply solutions when the executive board's objectives are at cross-purposes with the long-term strategies embedded in this methodology. Bolton hospital has shown what can be achieved when the whole organization, headed and supported by the CEO, work in unison.

After the second NHS lean healthcare forum in Birmingham last June, Dan Jones suggested that the next stage must include the primary NHS services, and only then would the true benefits of lean healthcare be realised. Regarding the 18-week time scale from GP request to hospital treatment set out by the government, Jones has challenged: "I think it could be done in 18 days and that is the target we should be aiming for."

Andrew Scotchmer, *a fellow of the Royal Statistical Society and member of the International Institute for business Analysis, is currently employed by the East Lancashire Hospitals NHS Trust and was responsible for initiating its lean implementation programme that was formally adopted in October 2006. Andrew may be contacted by email at: andrew.scotchmer@ntlworld.com.*

Appendix I

No Satisfaction at Toyota[*]

*What drives Toyota? The
presumption of imperfection—
and a distinctly American
refusal to accept it.*

From Fast Company *magazine, Issue 111,
December/January, Page 82. By Charles Fishman[†]*

Deep inside Toyota's (NYSE:TM) car factory in Georgetown, Kentucky, is the paint shop, where naked steel car bodies arrive to receive layers of coatings and colors before returning to the assembly line to have their interiors and engines installed. Every day, 2,000 Camrys, Avalons, and Solaras glide in to be painted one of a dozen colors by carefully programmed robots.

Georgetown's paint shop is vast and crowded, but in two places there are wide areas of open concrete floor, each the size of a basketball court. The story of how that floor space came to be cleared—

---

[*]*Author's note:* This appendix is not about healthcare. It is about the philosophy or zen that Toyota uses to keep improving every day. Toyota not only has the primary objective of producing the highest quality automobiles at the lowest prices, it also has the objective of relentlessly searching to find the most efficient processes to do so. Toyota is not just interested in making automobiles; it is interested in making great processes. It is this philosophy that healthcare providers need to adopt to continually improve healthcare quality and cost.

[†]Charles Fishman is a *Fast Company* senior writer and author of *The Wal-Mart Effect.*

tons of equipment dismantled and removed—is really the story of how Toyota has reshaped the U.S. car market.

It's the story of Toyota's genius: an insatiable competitiveness that would seem un-American were it not for all the Americans making it happen. Toyota's competitiveness is quiet, internal, self-critical. It is rooted in an institutional obsession with improvement that Toyota manages to instill in each one of its workers, a pervasive lack of complacency with whatever was accomplished yesterday.

The result is a startling contrast to the car business. At a time when the traditional Big Three are struggling, Toyota is thriving. Just this year, Ford (NYSE:F) and GM (NYSE:GM) have terminated 46,000 North American employees. Together, they have announced the closing of 26 North American factories over the next five years. Toyota has never closed a North American factory; it will open a new one in Texas this fall and another in Ontario in 2008. Detroit isn't being bested by imports: 60% of the cars Toyota sells in North America are made here.

Toyota doesn't have corporate convulsions, and it never has. It restructures a little bit every work shift. That's what the open space in the Georgetown paint shop is all about.

Chad Buckner helped clear the space. Buckner, 35, has a soft Southern accent and an air of helpfulness. He is an engineering manager in the painting department, where he arrived straight out of the University of Kentucky 13 years ago. His whole career has been spent at Toyota.

As recently as 2004, a car body spent 10 hours in painting. Robots did much of the work, then as now, but they were supplied with paint through long hoses from storage tanks. "If we were painting a car red, before we could paint the next car white, we had to stop, flush the red paint out of the lines and the applicator tip, and reload the next color," Buckner says. Georgetown literally threw away 30% of the pricey car paint it bought, cleaning it out of equipment and supply hoses when switching colors.

Now, each painting robot, eight per car, selects a paint cylinder the size of a large water bottle. A whirling disk at the end of the robot arm flings out a mist of top-coat paint. When a car is painted—it takes just seconds—the paint cartridge is set back down, and a freshly filled cartridge is selected by each robot.

No hoses need to be flushed. There is no cleaning between cars. All the paint is in the cartridges, which are refilled automatically from reservoirs. Cars don't need to be batched by color—a system that saved paint but caused constant delays. Cars now spend 8 hours in paint, instead of 10. The paint shop at any moment holds 25% fewer cars than it used to. Wasted paint? Practically zero. What used to require 100 gallons now takes 70.

The benefits ripple out. Not only does Georgetown use less paint, it also buys less cleaning solvent and has dramatically reduced disposal costs for both. Together with new programming to make the robots paint more quickly, Buckner's group has increased the efficiency of its car-wash-sized paint booths from 33 cars an hour to 50.

"We're getting the same volume with two booths that we used to get with three," Buckner says. "So we shut down one of the booths." If you want to trim your energy bill, try unplugging an oven big enough to bake 25 cars. Workers dismantled Top Coat Booth C, leaving the open floor space available for some future task.

So what do Buckner and his crew do with a triumphant operational improvement like that? By way of an answer, he walks to the second area of open space, where the sealer-application robots used to sit. They've been consolidated, too. Buckner points to another undercoating booth that the engineering staff is now working to eliminate.

Indeed, shutting down Top Coat Booth C liberated a handful of maintenance engineers—who turned their attention to accelerating the next round of changes. Success, in that way, becomes the platform for further improvement. By the end of this year, Buckner and his team hope to have cut almost in half the amount of floor space the paint shop needs—all while continuing to paint 2,000 cars a day.

For Buckner, the paint-shop improvements aren't "projects" or "initiatives." They are the work, his work, every day, every week. That's one of the subtle but distinctive characteristics of a Toyota factory. The supervisors and managers aren't "bosses" in any traditional American sense. Their job is to find ways to do the work better: more efficiently, more effectively.

"We're all incredibly proud of what we've accomplished," says Buckner, a little puzzled that his attitude might be considered unusual. "But you don't stop. You don't stop. There's no reason to be satisfied."

THE PROCESS PROCESS

What is so striking about Toyota's Georgetown factory is, in fact, that it only looks like a car factory. It's really a big brain—a kind of laboratory focused on a single mission: not how to make cars, but how to make cars better. The cars it does make—one every 27 seconds—are in a sense just a by-product of the larger mission. Better cars, sure; but really, better ways to make cars. It's not just the product, it's the process.

The process is, in fact, paramount—so important that "Toyota also has a process for teaching you how to improve the process," says Steven J. Spear, a senior lecturer at MIT who has studied Toyota for more than a decade. The work is really threefold: making cars, making cars better, and teaching everyone how to make cars better. At its Olympian best, Toyota adds one more level: It is always looking to improve the process by which it improves all the other processes.

There's a certain Zen sensibility to that—but also a relentlessly capitalistic, tenaciously competitive quality. If your factory is just making cars, once a day the whistle blows and it's quitting time, no more cars to make that day. If your factory is making a new way to make cars, the whistle never blows, you're never done.

Without fanfare, in fact, Toyota is confounding conventional wisdom about U.S. manufacturing. Toyota isn't outsourcing; it's creating jobs in the United States. It isn't having trouble manufacturing complicated products here—it's opening factories as quickly as its systems and quality standards allow. It's offering union wages and good health insurance (to avoid being unionized), and selling the products its American workers make to Americans, profitably and more inexpensively than its U.S. competitors.

So put aside everything you think you know about the current state of the car business in the United States. Sure, Toyota enjoys some structural advantages in the form of lower health care and pension costs. But the real reason it is thriving is because of people like Chad Buckner saying, "There's no reason to be satisfied." It's not just the way Toyota makes cars—it's the way Toyota thinks about making cars.

That thinking is hardly novel: Lean manufacturing and continuous improvement have been around for more than a quarter-century.

But the incessant, almost mindless repetition of those phrases camouflages the real power behind the ideas. Continuous improvement is tectonic. By constantly questioning how you do things, by constantly tweaking, you don't outflank your competition next quarter. You outflank them next decade.

Toyota is far from infallible, of course. In the past two years, recalls for quality and safety problems have spiked dramatically—evidence of the strain that rapid growth puts on even the best systems. But those quality issues have seized the attention of Toyota's senior management. In the larger arena, when the strategy isn't to build cars but to build cars better, you create perpetual competitive advantage. By the time you best your competitors, they aren't just a bit behind you, in need of a reorganization and a sales surge to regain the lead. They are a decade behind. They just don't realize it.

THE STORY OF THE TOTES

The Toyota factory in Georgetown sits on a piece of green ground as flat as a table. The factory itself is low, yet so large it stretches to the horizon, no matter what side you approach it from. There's space inside to play 100 football games, with room for fans on the sidelines. A network of heavily trafficked streets runs through the place, with travel lanes in each direction.

Cars are the most complicated objects most people use routinely; to watch cars get made is to pull back the curtain on raw human ingenuity. At Georgetown, that ingenuity often appears in unexpected, and unexpectedly simple, ways.

Howard Artrip, 45, is standing at the assembly line alongside a rack of blue plastic totes filled with sun visors and seat belts. Just beyond Artrip and the rack of totes, a line of Camrys and Avalons pass by, freshly painted but hollow—no engines, no dashboards, no seats.

Artrip, a manager in the assembly area, is telling the story of how the totes—ordinary Rubbermaid carryalls—solved a decision-making problem. "There used to be eight racks of parts here," he says. The racks crowded the workstation, giving the worker ready access to all possible parts. The operator would eyeball the car coming up the line, step to the racks of visors and seat belts, and, says

Artrip, "grab the right parts and run to the car." He or she would step into the slowly advancing car, bolt belts and visors in place, step back onto the factory floor—and do it again. All in 55 seconds, the unvarying time each slowly moving car spends at each workstation.

The problem was, there were 12 possible combinations of sun visors and nine variations of seat belts. So just deciding which parts to snatch had become a job in itself. In every shift, 500 cars passed the racks, each car needing four specific parts: 2,000 opportunities to make an error. Even with 99% perfection, five cars per shift got the wrong sun visors or seat belts. The job—installing parts—had become cluttered with meaningless decision making.

So a team of assembly employees made a real decision. Don't make the worker pick the parts; let him focus on installing them. The idea seems obvious in retrospect: Deliver a kit of presorted visors and seat belts—one kit per car, each containing exactly the right parts. The team applied the simplest technology available, the blue Rubbermaid caddy. "We went just down the road to Wal-Mart and bought them," Artrip says. Now, the line worker doesn't have to make any decisions at all. Just grab the handle of the blue tote like a lunch pail and step into the car.

Media accounts often report that a typical Toyota assembly line in the United States makes thousands of operational changes in the course of a single year. That number is not just large, it's arresting, it's mind-boggling. How much have you changed your work routine in the past decade? Toyota's line employees change the way they work dozens of times a year.

In the case of the blue tote, the change came out of a routine analysis of dozens of assembly-line jobs at Georgetown. When the simplification effort started three years ago, Artrip's team found 44 jobs where assemblers had to make 1 or 2 decisions as they installed parts. They found 23 workstations that required between 7 and 11 decisions.

Any jobs requiring 7 to 11 decisions in 55 seconds were going to cause problems. So dozens of jobs incurred small changes—grab the blue tote instead of choosing individual parts. Now, 85 line jobs require just 1 or 2 decisions. Not a single job requires 7 or more decisions. The work is easier, the results are better.

This is exactly the kind of work Artrip has spent more than half his career at Toyota doing: looking for ways to make the assembly line faster, simpler, safer—ways to make it easier to do the work perfectly. Continuous improvement is not some add-on to the real work, it isn't some special project Artrip has to do on top of his routine responsibilities, nor is he a guy who parachutes into the assembly line from an engineering building somewhere else. It is what he comes to the factory every day thinking about. It isn't exhausting, it's exhilarating.

Artrip has been at Georgetown for 19 years. The way he does his work is so compelling it has become part of his personal life. "When I'm mowing the grass, I'm thinking about the best way to do it. I'm trying different turns to see if I can do it faster," he says. He has analyzed his morning routine. "I do the same standardized work in the shower every morning. I have to get here at 6 a.m., and I know it takes 19 minutes, including walking into the plant." He smiles. "I've maximized my sleep time."

PROBLEMS FIRST

James Wiseman remembers the moment he realized that Toyota wasn't just another workplace but a different way of thinking about work. Before joining the company, he had been a factory manager, first for a swimsuit maker, then for a steel-tubing manufacturer. He joined Toyota's still-new Georgetown plant in October 1989 as manager of community relations. Today, he's vice president of corporate affairs for all of Toyota manufacturing in North America.

At the swimsuit factory and the tube factory, "there was always a lot of looking for the silver bullet," Wiseman says, "looking for the big, dramatic improvement. And I had the attitude that when you achieved something, you achieved it. You enjoyed it." He was steeped in the American business culture of not admitting, or even discussing, problems in settings like meetings.

In Wiseman's early days, Georgetown was run by Fujio Cho, now the chairman of Toyota worldwide. Every Friday, there was a senior staff meeting. "I started out going in there and reporting some of my little successes," says Wiseman. "One Friday, I gave a report of an activity we'd been doing"—planning the announcement of a plant expansion—"and I spoke very positively about it, I bragged a little. After two or three minutes, I sat down."

"And Mr. Cho kind of looked at me. I could see he was puzzled. He said, 'Jim-san. We all know you are a good manager, otherwise we would not have hired you. But please talk to us about your problems so we can all work on them together.' "

Wiseman says it was like a lightning bolt. "Even with projects that had been a general success, we would ask, 'What didn't go well so we can make it better?' " At Toyota, Wiseman says, "I have come to understand what they mean when I hear the phrase, 'Problems first.' "

It's another cliché that is powerful if you take it seriously: You can't solve problems unless you admit them. At Toyota, there is a presumption of imperfection. Perfection is a fine goal, but improvement is much more realistic, much more human. Not a 15% improvement by the end of the quarter, a 1% improvement by the end of the month.

The challenge, of course, is to make the rhetoric real, to make the presumption of imperfection integral to how people think and work. Pete Gritton knows better than most how that happens; he and his staff have hired all the Kentuckians who work at Toyota Georgetown. He's vice president of HR and administration for Georgetown, and vice president of HR for Toyota manufacturing in North America.

"We want people to be problem solvers," Gritton says. "Because every time there's a problem, we don't send out some guy in a white shirt with a clipboard." New hires—10% of job applicants make it through screening tests that include a team-building exercise—are immersed in Toyota's process for process improvement. There are daily work-group meetings, a written suggestion program, and longer-term problem-solving teams. But everything is grounded in two hard realities.

First, of course, "we have to make 2,000 cars a day. We can't vote about how to make each one," Gritton says. "We can't stop every few minutes and change the process." And then there is the most basic rule, the reason "continuous improvement" is not a matter of character or national culture or willpower, but is itself a kind of assembly line. "The rule here is that improving something starts after understanding the standard—understanding how we do it now," Gritton says. "If you don't understand what you're trying to improve, how do you know that your suggestion is an improvement?"

No one at Toyota Georgetown can talk about his work without explaining how it has just changed, or is about to change. Chris

Gentry, a supervisor for instrument-panel assembly, is showing how his area is about to be redesigned. It was set up just this year to handle the 2007 Camry—but after working with it for most of a year, workers now see inefficiencies. Some work will be moved back to an area where kits are assembled; some movement of parts can be off-loaded to seven newly built transport robots. Two jobs will be eliminated and the workers redeployed elsewhere; 18 seconds can be shaved from the assembly process.

"We set it up for the model change," says Gentry. "Now we'll fix it. We standardized it, now we're improving it." It's not the instrument panel—it's the way you make the instrument panel.

In the 2007 Camry, there is a tiny change that drivers won't notice. The Camry's radiator support bar—a brace of steel running across the lower front of the engine compartment—isn't installed when the body is first made. It used to be, but it blocked access to the engine compartment. Workers had to stretch and lean in to install engine wiring and components. With the bar's installation held out until near the end of assembly, workers simply step into the engine compartment and get right up close to their work. That idea ricocheted from the plant floor in Georgetown, up to Toyota's design team, and then out to Camry assembly plants around the world.

Once you see how woven into the work improving the work is, each particular improvement seem less interesting. What's interesting is to compare how they think about work at Georgetown with everywhere else. How come the checkout lines at Wal-Mart never get shorter? How come the customer service of your cell-phone company never improves, year after year? How come my PC gets harder to operate with each software upgrade? How come I don't know how many minutes it takes me to get from my doorstep to my office, so I can maximize my sleep?

It's almost as if Toyota people see the world with special four-dimensional glasses; the rest of us are stuck in 2-D.

IN THE END, THERE IS NO END

Lots of companies have tried to learn and use the methods that Toyota has refined into a routine, a science, a way of being and thinking. Not least among those are...GM, Ford, and Chrysler

(NYSE:DCX). For more than 20 years, in fact, Toyota and GM have operated a car factory together in California—the NUMMI project—that has allowed GM to study Toyota's methods up close.

And the Big Three have each gotten better at making cars: In the past decade, GM and Chrysler have cut by one-third the hours they need to assemble a car. But they all still trail Toyota. No one knows that better than GM. "We've made a whole lot of progress," says Dan Flores, a spokesman for GM's North American manufacturing operations—much of it by learning directly from Toyota. "Transforming a company the size of GM is a daunting task. The culture of the plants doesn't change overnight. But there has been a cultural change in the company—and that change continues."

Typically, though, the Big Three take an all-too-American approach to the idea of improvement. It's episodic, it's goal-oriented, it's something special—it's a pale imitation of the approach at Georgetown. "If you go to the Big Three, you'd find improvement projects just like you'd find at Georgetown," says Jeffrey Liker, a professor of engineering at the University of Michigan and author of *The Toyota Way*, a classic exploration of Toyota's methods. "But they would be led by some kind of engineering group, or a Six Sigma black belt, or a lean-manufacturing guru of some kind.

"They might even do as good a job as they did at Georgetown. But here's the thing. Then they'd turn that project into a PowerPoint. They'd present it at every place in the whole company. They'd say, 'Look what we did!' In a year, that happens a couple of times in a whole plant for the Big Three. And it would get all kinds of publicity in the company.

"Toyota," Liker says, "is doing it in every single department, every single day. They're doing it on their own"—no black belts—" and they're doing it regularly, not just once."

So you can buy the books, you can hire the consultants, you can implement the program, you can preach business transformation— and you can eventually run out of energy, lose enthusiasm, be puzzled over why the program failed to catch fire and transform your business, put the fat binders on a conference-room shelf, and go back to business as usual.

What happens every day at Georgetown, and throughout Toyota, is teachable and learnable. But it's not a set of goals, because goals mean there's a finish line, and there is no finish line. It's not something you can implement, because it's not a checklist of improvements. It's a way of looking at the world. You simply can't lose interest in it, shrug, and give up—any more than you can lose interest in your own future.

"People who join Toyota from other companies, it's a big shift for them," says John Shook, a faculty member at the University of Michigan, a former Toyota manufacturing employee and a widely regarded consultant on how to use Toyota's ideas at other companies. "They kind of don't get it for a while." They do what all American managers do—they keep trying to make their management objectives. "They're moving forward, they're improving, and they're looking for a plateau. As long as you're looking for that plateau, it seems like a constant struggle. It's difficult. If you're looking for a plateau, you're going to be frustrated. There is no 'solution.'"

Even working at Toyota, you need that moment of Zen.

"Once you realize that it's the process itself—that you're not seeking a plateau—you can relax. Doing the task and doing the task better become one and the same thing," Shook says. "This is what it means to come to work."

- Toyota's sales gain in 2005 from three years before: **34%**

- Its profit per car: **$1,587**

- Share of cars it sells in North America that are made here: **60%**

Notes

Chapter 1

1. See "Hospital Bills Spin Out of Control" at http://usatoday.com/money/industries/health/2004-04-13-rising-hospital-costs_x.htm, http://www.usatoday.com/money/industries/health/2003-09-09-healthcare-costs_x.htm, and http://www.hospitalconnect.com/hret/publications/content/NewRelease.pdf.
2. William J. Latzko and David M. Saunders, *Four Days with Dr. Deming* (Reading, MA: Addison Wesley, 1995): 131.
3. See http://www.uaw.org/barg/03/barg02.cfm.
4. See http://www.aier.org/2004pubs/RR01.pdf, "American Institute for Economic Research," *Research Reports* 71, no. 1 (2004).
5. Lucette Lagnado, "California Hospitals Open Book, Showing Huge Price Differences," *Wall Street Journal* (December 27, 2004): A1 and A6. Also available at http://www.trinity.edu/eschumac/HCAI5313/WSJ_com%20-%20California%20Hospitals%20Open%20Books,%20Showing%20Huge%20Price%20Differences.htm or http://suttercorporatewatch.org/news/WSJ12-27-04.pdf.
6. You may read this enlightening report at: http://s57.advocateoffice.com/vertical/Sites/%7B56490583-267C-4278-BC56-A7128CE248A8%7D/uploads/%7B374CBAD9-740D-48BC-8536-92ECD76D1444%7D.PDF
7. See http://jec.senate.gov/Documents/Reports/healthinsurance2006.pdf.

8. David U. Himmelstein, Elizabeth Warren, Deborah Thorne, and Steffie Woolhandler, "Illness and Injury As Contributors to Bankruptcy," *Health Affairs* (February 2, 2005).

9. Melissa Jacoby et. al., "Rethinking the Debates over Health Care Financing: Evidence from the Bankruptcy Courts," *New York University Law Review* 76, no. 2 (May 2001).

10. U.S. Department of Labor Statistics, "Occupational Employment Projections to 2014," *Monthly Labor Review* (November 2005).

11. See http://www.commerce.gov/DOC_MFG_Report_Complete.pdf.

12. See www.Lean.org.

13. James Womack and Dan Jones, *Lean Thinking* (New York: Simon & Schuster, 1996).

14. See http://www.everybodyinnobodyout.org.

15. See http://www.usatoday.com/money/industries/health/2004-09-29-nonprofit-salaries_x.htm?POE=click-refer.

16. See http://www.everybodyinnobodyout.org.

17. Jennifer Steinhauer, "California Plan for Healthcare Would Cover All," *New York Times* (January 9, 2007).

18. Steffie Woolhandler, MD, "Cost of Health Care Administration in the United States and Canada," *New England Journal of Medicine* 349, no. 8 (August 21, 2003): 768–75.

19. For an in-depth discussion of administrative costs and waste, see David U. Himmelstein, Steffie Woolhandler, and Sidney M. Wolfe, "The Cost to the Nation, the States and the District of Columbia, with State-Specific Estimates of Potential Savings," Public Citizen Health Research Group (http://www.citizen.org/publications/release.cfm?ID=7271). This article also contains a good discussion of the advantages of single-payer systems such as the Canadian healthcare system.

20. See http://www.cms.hhs.gov.

21. See http://www.who.int.

22. See http://www.intelihealth.com/IH/ihtIH/WSMST000/333/8896/377730.html.

23. Gerard Anderson, "Comparing Health System Performance in OECD Countries," *Health Affairs* 20, no. 3 (May/June 2001): 219–32.

24. The most recent complete comparative data analyses for infant mortality rates are from 2003, according to the National Center for Health Statistics, "Preventing Infant Mortality," HHS Fact Sheet, U.S. Department of Health and Human Services, January 13, 2006.

25. See http://www.mbgh.org.

26. Elizabeth A. McGlynn, Steven M. Asch, John Adams, Joan Keesey, Jennifer Hicks, and Alison DeCristofaro, "The Quality of Health Care

Delivered to Adults in the United States," *New England Journal of Medicine 348*:26 (June 26, 2003), 2635-2645. See also http://www.ripolicyanalysis.org/QualityofCareinUS.pdf or http://www.nejm.org.

27. Linda T. Kohn, Janet M. Corrigan, and Molla S. Donaldson, Editors, *To Err Is Human: Building a Safer Health System* (Washington, DC: National Academies Press, 2000).

28. *Ibid.*

29. Robin E. McDermott, *The Basics of FMEA* (Portland, OR: Productivity Press, 1996).

30. See http://www.programbusiness.com/NewsFinance/ ArticleDetail.asp?artID=1372 and http://www.usatoday.com/ money/industries/health/2004-04-12-hospital-coverside_x.htm.

31. For another good presentation of how to monitor community health status indicators, see http://www.doh.state.fl.us/family/mch/docs/ fy2003/fy2003support1.pdf.

Chapter 3

1. For discussions of payer and financing systems and macro healthcare delivery issues, you may refer to John P. Geyman, "The Corporate Transformation of Medicine and Its Impact on Costs and Access to Care" *Journal of the American Board of Family Practice* 16, no. 5 (September–October 2003): 443–54 at http://www.jabfp.org/cgi/ content/full/16/5/443 or to articles by Marcia Angell or George D. Lundberg, *Severed Trust* (New York: Basic Books, 2000).

2. James Womack's and John Shook's 2006 presentation "Lean Management and the Role of Lean Leadership" may be viewed at http://www.lean.org/Events/WatchWebinar.cfm.

3. See the "Psychology of Change Management" in *The McKinsey Quarterly* http://www.focusedperformance.com/2003_10_01_blarch .html#106518483109148038.

4. For more on queuing models, see this page at the University of Windsor Ontario http://www2.uwindsor.ca/~hlynka/queue.html. IHI.org also presents numerous queuing resources at http://www. ihi.org/ihi/search/searchresults.aspx?searchterm=queuing&searchtype =basic&Start+Search.x=0&Start+Search.y=0.

5. For an example of how nationally the recognized SSM Healthcare of St. Louis, MO, uses a graphical method to monitor key indicators, see section seven of their winning Baldrige National Quality Award application at http://baldrige.nist.gov/PDF_files/ SSM_Application_Summary.pdf. Another graphical scorecard

example from Saint Luke's Hospital of Kansas City, MO, may
be seen in section 7 at http://www.mqa.org/pdf/SLHcat7.pdf.
St. Luke's is the first healthcare organization to win the prestigious
Missouri Quality Award and has since become the first three-time
recipient of it.

6. See http://www.nummi.com/co_info.html.

7. This 5S example may also be found online at the Pittsburgh Regional
Healthcare Initiative PRHI Web site within the December 2003
newsletter, http://prhi.org/newsletters.cfm. The Pittsburgh Regional
Healthcare Initiative (http://www.prhi.org) contains many
improvement ideas that may be replicated elsewhere.

8. Taiichi Ohno, *Toyota Production System: Beyond Large-Scale
Production* (Cambridge, MA: Productivity Press, 1988): 41.

9. Christine Tierney, "Big 3 Still Lagging Japan," *Detroit News*
(February 22, 2004)

10. See "To Fix Health Care, Hospitals Take Tips from Factory Floor,"
Wall Street Journal (April 9, 2004) at http://www.ihaonline.org/
frimailing/2004/2004%20Enclosures/NS4-9-04.pdf.

11. James Womack, *The Machine That Changed the World: The Story of
Lean Production* (New York: Harper Perennial, 1991): 62.

12. Ohno, *Toyota Production System: Beyond Large-Scale Production*,
27, 30.

13. Kiyoshi Suzaki, *The New Manufacturing Challenge: Techniques for
Continuous Improvement* (New York: The Free Press, 1987): 17.

14. Neil Swideg, "The Revolutionary," *Boston Globe Magazine* (January
4, 2004).

15. *Technology Law Newsletter* (Spring 2003), available at
http://www.computerbar.org.

16. See http://www.websense.com and its competitors.

17. Ohno, *Toyota Production System*, 130.

18. See http://prhi.org/newsletters.cfm. The online article was written
with the help of PRHI communications director Naida Grunden. The
PRHI Web site, http://www.prhi.org, contains numerous improvement
examples that may be replicated by other healthcare providers.

19. Eliyahu M. Goldratt, *The Goal*, Third Edition (Great Barrington, MA:
North River Press, 2004).

20. See http://www.asq.org/health/docs/levett-iowa-the-physician
-executive.pdf.

21. See http://news.yahoo.com/news?tmpl=story&u=/ap/20040604/
ap_on_he_me/doctor_visits_1.

22. The past winners of the Baldrige award in healthcare are: In 2002,
Franciscan Sisters of Mary Healthcare (SSMHC) in St. Louis,

Missouri; in 2003, St. Luke's Hospital in Kansas City, Missouri and Baptist Hospital in Pensacola, Florida; in 2004, Robert Wood Johnson University Hospital in Hamilton, New Jersey; in 2005, Bronson Methodist Hospital in Kalamazoo, Michigan; and in 2006, North Mississippi Medical Center in Tupelo, Mississippi.

24. To learn more, please see http://baldrige.nist.gov/index.html and http://www.nist.gov/public_affairs/releases/ssmhealth.htm and http://www.ssmhc.com/internet/home/ssmcorp.nsf.

25. See http://www.ebaptisthealthcare.org/BaptistHospital/ and http://www.startribune.com/storics/308/4014401.html.

Chapter 5

1. Please see http://www.ncqa.org/Communications/News/ SOHC_2006.htm or http://www.unitedwaymc.org/media/ LIFE-Health.pdf.

Appendix D

Reprinted from *Clinics in Laboratory Medicine,* 24(4), Condel, Sharbaugh, and Raab, "Error-Free Pathology: Apply Lean Methods to Anatomic Pathology," pp. 865–99, copyright 2004, with permission from Elsevier.

1. J. Liker, *The Toyota Way: 14 Management Principles from the World's Greatest Manufacturer* (New York: McGraw-Hill, 2004).
2. T. Ohno, *Toyota Production System: Beyond Large-Scale Production* (Cambridge, MA: Productivity Press, 1988).
3. H. Johnson and A. Broms, *Profit Beyond Measure: Extraordinary Results Through Attention to Work and People* (New York: The Free Press, 2000).
4. S. Spear and K. Bowen, *Decoding the DNA of the Toyota Production System* (Harvard Business Press, 1999).
5. K. Mishina and K. Takeda, *Toyota Motor Manufacturing, USA, Inc.* (Harvard Business School, 1992).
6. Institute of Medicine, *To Err Is Human: Building a Safer Health System* (Washington, DC: National Academy Press, 1999).
7. Pittsburgh Regional Healthcare Initiative Web site. Available at: http://www.prhi.org. Accessed March 2004.
8. K. Feinstein, N. Grunden, and E. Harrison, "A Region Addresses Patient Safety" *American Journal of Infection Control* 30, no. 4 (2002): 248–51.
9. Pittsburgh Regional Healthcare Initiative. *Perfecting Patient Care System Educational Materials* (Pittsburgh: PRHI, 2002).

Apppendix G

1. John P. Burke, "Infection Control—A Problem for Patient Safety," *New England Journal of Medicine* (February 2003); William R. Jarvis, "Infection Control and Changing Health-Care Delivery Systems," *Emerging Infectious Diseases* (March–April 2001); Robert A. Weinstein, "Nosocomial Infection Update," *Emerging Infectious Diseases* (July–September 1998).

Bibliography

Berk, Joseph, and Susan Berk. *Total Quality Management: Implementing Continuous Improvement*. New York: Sterling Publishing, 1993.

Bodenstab, Charles J. *A New Era in Inventory Management for the Distribution Industry*. Minneapolis, MN: Hilta Press, 1993.

Carey, Raymond G. *Measuring Quality Improvement in Healthcare—A Guide to Statistical Process Control Applications*. New York: Quality Resources, 1995.

CC-M Productions, *How Hospitals Heal Themselves*, DVD video report for Public Television, 2006, available from www.managementwisdom.com, Tel 800-453-6280.

Crosby, Philip B. *Quality Is Free: The Art of Making Quality Certain*. New York: Mentor, 1980.

Dillon, Andrew P., trans. *The Sayings of Shigeo Shingo: Key Strategies for Plant Improvement*. Cambridge, MA: Productivity Press, 1985.

Dobyns, Lloyd. *Thinking About Quality: Progress, Wisdom, and the Deming Philosophy*. New York: Times Books, Random House, 1994.

Feld, William M. *Lean Manufacturing Tools, Techniques, and How to Use Them*. Boca Raton, FL: The St. Lucie Press, 2001.

Fisher, Dennis. *The Just-in-Time Self Test*. Chicago: Irwin Professional Publishing, 1995.

Fiume O., Cunningham J. E. *Real Numbers: Management Accounting in a Lean Organization*. Managing Times Press, 2003.

George, Michael L. *Lean Six Sigma for Service*. New York: McGraw-Hill, 2003.

Gross, John M. *Kanban Made Simple*. New York: AMACOM American Management Association, 2003.

Henderson, Bruce A. *Lean Transformation: How to Change Your Business into a Lean Enterprise.* Richmond, VA: The Oaklea Press, 1999.

Hines, Peter. *Value Stream Management.* Harlow, England and Reading, MA: Prentice Hall, 2000.

Hirano, Hiroyuki. *5S for Operators: 5 Pillars of the Visual Workplace.* Portland, OR: Productivity Press, 1996.

Japan Management Association. *Kanban: Just-in-Time at Toyota.* Portland, OR: Productivity Press, 1985.

Johnson, H. *Profit Beyond Measure: Extraordinary Results through Attention to Work and People.* New York: The Free Press, 2000.

Kobayashi, Iwao. *20 Keys to Workplace Improvement.* Cambridge, MA: Productivity Press, 1988.

Lamprecht, James L. *ISO 9000: Preparing for Registration.* Milwaukee: ASQC Quality Press, 1992.

Latzko, William J. *Four Days with Dr. Deming.* Reading, MA: Addison-Wesley, 1995.

Liker, Jeffrey K. *The Toyota Way: 14 Management Principles from the World's Greatest Manufacturer.* New York: McGraw-Hill, 2004.

Lundberg, George D., MD. *Severed Trust: Why American Medicine Hasn't Been Fixed.* New York: Basic Books, Perseus Books Group, 2000.

McDermott, Robin E. *The Basics of FMEA: Failure Mode and Effects Analysis.* Portland, OR: Productivity Press, 1996.

Mears, Peter. *Quality Improvement Tools & Techniques.* New York: McGraw-Hill, 1995.

Nauman, Earl, and Steven H. Hoisington. *Customer Centered Six Sigma.* Milwaukee: ASQ Quality Press, 2001.

Ohno, Taiichi. *Toyota Production System: Beyond Large-Scale Production.* Cambridge, MA: Productivity Press, 1988.

Pande, Pete. *What Is Six Sigma?* New York: McGraw-Hill, 2002.

Rother M., Shook J., Womack J. P., Jones D. T. *Learning to See.* Boston: Lean Enterprise Institute; Version 1.3, 2003.

Salvendy, Gavriel, ed. *Handbook of Industrial Engineering.* New York: John Wiley & Sons, 2001.

Sandras, William A. Jr. *Just-in-Time: Making It Happen.* Essex Junction, VT: Oliver Wight Limited Publications, 1989.

Savary, Louis M., and Clare Crawford-Mason, *The Nun and the Bureaucrat*, Washington, DC, CC-M Productions, 2006.

Schonberger, Richard J. *Japanese Manufacturing Techniques: Nine Hidden Lessons in Simplicity.* New York: The Free Press, 1982.

Slater, Robert. *29 Leadership Secrets from Jack Welch.* New York: McGraw-Hill, 2003.

Spear S. J. *Learning to lead at Toyota.* Harvard Business Review. 2004 May;82(5):78–86, 151.

Suzaki, Kiyoshi. *The New Manufacturing Challenge: Techniques for Continuous Improvement.* New York: The Free Press, 1987.

―――. *The New Shop Floor Management: Empowering People for Continuous Improvement* (New York: The Free Press, 1993.

To Err Is Human: Building a Safer Health System. Washington, DC: National Acedemy Press, 1999.

White House Domestic Policy Council. *The President's Health Security Plan.* New York: Times Books, Random House, 1993.

Womack, James P. *The Machine That Changed the World: The Story of Lean Production.* New York: Harper Perennial, 1991.

Womack J. P., Jones D. T. *Lean Thinking: Banish Waste and Create Wealth in Your Corporation.* New York: Simon and Schuster, Inc.; 1996, Second Edition 2003.

Zandin, Kjell B., ed. *Maynard's Industrial Engineering Handbook.* New York: McGraw-Hill, 2001.

Glossary of Lean Terms*

5–S: Sort, Simplify, Sweep, Standardize, Self-Discipline: a visually-oriented system for organizing the workplace to minimize the waste of time.

5 why's: When an error or defect occurs, it's important to ask "Why?" five times to get to the true root cause of the problem. Otherwise one may try to correct a symptom as opposed to correcting the real cause.

Adequate: In value stream mapping, the capacity for any given step in a process is adequate if the process is not delayed at that step.

Autonomation: Machines and equipment are built with "human intelligence" and are able to detect and prevent defects. Machines stop autonomously when defects are detected, asking for help. Autonomation was pioneered by Sakichi Toyoda with the invention of automatic looms that stopped when a thread broke, allowing an operator to manage many looms without risk of producing large amounts of defective cloth.

---

*Note that much of this glossary first appeared in the paper "Going Lean in Healthcare." in Appendix E.

Autonomation, also known as jidoka, is a pillar of the Toyota Production System.

Available: In value stream mapping, a step in a process is available if it produces the desired output, not just the desired quality, every time.

Batch-and-queue: The mass-production practice of making large lots of a part then sending the batch to wait in the queue before the next operation in the production process. Contrast with single-piece flow.

Capable: In value stream mapping, a step in a process is capable if it produces a good result every time.

Cellular or flow: The aim of one-piece flow is to physically link and arrange process steps into the most efficient combination, thus maximizing value added content while minimizing waste. Cellular flow allows one or a few cross-trained workers to perform all the functions in a well arranged work cell and to share duties.

Continuous level flow: Production continues at an optimal steady rate. It is desirable to level demand and the needed rate of production so that level flow is maintained without overburdening employees.

Cycle time: The time required for completing one step of a process.

Error proofing (poka yoke): Processes and equipment are designed to eliminate the possibility of an error from ever occurring. This prevents "accidents waiting to happen."

Flow: The progressive achievement of tasks along the value stream so that a product proceeds from design to launch, order to delivery, and raw materials into the hands of the customer with no stoppages, scrap, or backflows.

Heijunka: "production leveling." Averaging out demand over a set time period. This can be a challenge in a busy and unpredictable hospital environment.

Jidoka: a method for "building in quality." The empowerment of all staff to raise nonconformances when defects have occurred and to become involved in their solution.

Just-in-Time: A system for producing and delivering the right items at the right time in the right amounts. Just-in-Time approaches just-on-time when upstream activities occur minutes or seconds before downstream activities, so single-piece flow is possible. The key elements of Just-in-Time are flow, pull, standard work (with standard in-process inventories), and *takt* time.

Kaikaku: also termed a "kaizen blitz." Kaikaku is a rapid change to processes in order to improve the current system and receive immediate benefits. Often includes radical ideas that involve creative changes to the process. Takes place over a five-day workshop.

*Kaizen***:** Continuous, incremental improvement of an activity to create more value with less *muda*.

*Kanban***:** A signal, often a card attached to supplies or equipment that regulates pull by signaling upstream production and delivery.

Lead time: The total time a customer must wait to receive a product after requesting the product or service. In service sectors, it is the time from the beginning of the process to the end (e.g., from when a patient arrives until he or she leaves the hospital).

Muda: the Japanese term for waste. Taiichi Ohno described seven forms of waste: inventory, waiting, overproduction, unnecessary transporting, unnecessary movement, defects, and unnecessary possessing.

People distance: The distance staff must travel to accomplish their tasks.

Perfection: the ultimate goal where all four principles work in total harmony, mutually supportive, internally consistent.

Point of use storage (POUS): Supplies, equipment, and information, work standards, procedures, and policies are stored near the staff where they are needed.

Process capability and reducing variation: Processes are designed to produce consistently high-quality results with minimal variation or defects.

Product distance: The distance products must travel to meet the customers' needs.

Pull: A system of cascading production and delivery instructions from downstream to upstream activities in which nothing is produced by the upstream supplier until the downstream customer signals a need; the opposite of push.

Quality at the source: Inspection and process control are carried out by the front line staff doing the work so they are certain the patient or product passed to the next process is of acceptable quality. Providing quality at the source eliminates the waste of re-inspection and correction.

Quick changeover: The ability to change equipment and work areas (such as ORs) usually in minutes allows for more procedures using the same resources.

Set-up time: All time spent getting ready to add value (e.g., time preparing a room for an office visit).

Single-piece flow: A situation in which products proceed, one complete product at a time, through various operations in design, order-taking, and production, without interruptions, backflows or scrap. Contrast with batch-and-queue.

Standard work: A precise description of each work activity specifying cycle time, takt time, the work sequence of specific tasks for each team member, and the minimum inventory of parts on hand needed to conduct the activity.

Supplier development: Suppliers are treated as key partners to optimize overall results. A few key suppliers that deliver top performance are relied upon and cultivated.

Takt **time:** The available production time divided by the rate of customer demand. For example, if customers demand 240 widgets per day and the factory operates 480 minutes per day, *takt* time is two minutes. *Takt* time sets the pace of production to match the rate of customer demand and becomes the heartbeat of any lean system.

Throughput time: The time required for a product to proceed from concept to launch, order to delivery, or raw materials into the hands of the customer. This includes both processing and queue time.

Total productive maintenance (TPM): This lean equipment maintenance strategy maximizes overall equipment effectiveness. Many building blocks are interconnected and can be implemented in tandem. For example, 5S, visual controls, point of use storage, standardized work, streamlined layout, working in teams and autonomous maintenance (part of total productive maintenance) can all be components of a planned implementation effort.

Trystorm: To generate and quickly try ideas, or models of ideas, rather than simply discuss them, as in brainstorming.

Value: A capability provided to the customer at the right time at an appropriate price, as defined in each case by the customer.

Value stream: The specific activities required to design, order, and provide a specific product (or service)—from concept launch to order to delivery into the hands of the customer.

Value stream mapping: Identification of all the specific activities occurring along a value stream for a product or product family (or service).

Valuable: In value stream mapping, a step in a process is valuable if it creates value for the customer.

Visual workplace: All equipment, supplies, activities, and indicators are in view so everyone involved can understand the status of the system and the work processes at a glance. Equipment, instruments, and supplies are visibly stored in standard places. Work and workers remain visible so that the pace of work is clear.

Waste: Anything that does not add value to the final product or service, in the eyes of the customer; an activity the customer wouldn't want to pay for if they knew it was happening.

Index

A3 form, 48–49
administrative costs, 22–30, 130, 138
administrators, 52–54, 103–04
advanced diagnostics and treatment,
  68
Aetna, 28
Agency for Health Care Research and
  Quality, 166
Allegheny General Hospital, 245
Alukal, G., 213
ambiguity in hospital setting, 235–42
American Hospital Association
  (AHA), 140
anatomic pathology case study, 157–
  90
  continuous flow, 181–89
  cycle time data, 174–75
  demand data, 171–72
  evolution of lean, 158–59
  5S process, 175–80
  healthcare application, 165–66
  learning line, 167–75
  Toyota's lean enterprise, 159–65
andon board/cord, 84, 89–91, 163, 205
annual financial report, 66–67
annual quality report, 66–67
Appleby, J., 264
automaker benchmarks, 144
automation of processes, 122
autonomation, 221

Baldrige National Quality Award, 72,
  127–29

Baptist Health Care (BHC), 127–28
batch size reduction, 220
Bates, D. W., 236
benchmarking, 122–26
  benchmark values, 68
  healthcare organizations, 127–29
  McDonald's lessons, 125–26
  nonhealthcare organizations,
    124–26
  Wal-Mart's lessons, 123–25
Berwick, D., 21, 46, 103, 105, 132
Black, I., 259
board-approved strategic goal teams,
  65
Board of Directors, 65–66
bottlenecks, 110–12, 223
Bouché, B., 145
Bowen, K., 162, 171
brainstorming, 223, 225
Buckner, C., 268–69, 270
Bush, George W., 7, 16
business value added (BVA), 48, 59,
  116–17
buy-in, 55–56
Byrne, A. P., 191

Caldwell, P., 161
California Healthcare Association, 11
"California Hospitals Open Books,
  Showing Hugh Price
  Differences" (Lagnado), 10
California Plan for Healthcare (2007),
  26

Canadian Universal Healthcare
    System, 23–27
Care for Ohio, 11–12
Caremark Rx, Inc., 28
cellular flow, 221
Census Bureau, 13
Centers for Disease Control and
    Prevention (CDC), 230–31
Centers for Medicare and Medicaid
    Services, 30, 237
Chalice, R., 213
change management, 53, 55–56, 136,
    218, 242–45, 253–55
changeover improvement process,
    222–23
charity care standards, 11
chief executive officers (CEOs),
    22–27
Children's Hospital and Regional
    Medical Center Emergency
    Department Patient Flow—
    Rapid Process Improvement
    (RPI), 145–50
chosen solution (*nemawashi*), 80
committees/task forces, 101
Commonwealth Fund, 13–14
communication, 79, 148, 225
Condel, J., 110, 157
Conemaugh Health System, 252
consumer price index (CPI), 8
continuous flow, 50, 137, 160–62,
    222, 263
    anatomic pathology, 181–89
    bottlenecks and, 110–12
    implementation/maintaining,
        113–14
continuous improvement teams, 218
continuous quality improvement
    (CQI), past failures of, 38–39
control board (*andon*), 84, 89–91, 163,
    205
core processes, 38–50, 59–60, 116–17
Corrigan, J. M., 232
cost control, 15
cost improvements, organizational
    structure for, 77
cost per case mix indexed (CMI)
    adjusted patient discharge, 22,
    57, 68
Crosby, P., 46, 72

cross-training, 75
culture, 91, 195–96, 198
cycle time, 84, 117–18, 174–75

"Decoding the DNA of the Toyota
    Production System" (Spear and
    Bowen), 162
defects and reworks, 88–93, 181, 205,
    215, 221
delays, 50, 93–94, 215
Deming, W. Edwards, 5, 41, 46, 72,
    160–61; 192
demonstration site, 139–40
departmental scorecard (example), 64
direct patient value-added employees,
    104
discharge planners, 104
DMAIC steps (define, measure,
    analyze, improve, and control),
    92, 216
do-it groups (DIGS), 66
documentation of standardized
    processes, 112–13
Donaldson, M. S., 232
downsizing, 41
Drucker, P., 41, 46
Dunphy, M., 145
Durenberger, D., 12

email, 108
Emerson, J., 11
employees
    communication with, 79, 148, 225
    easing change transition, 55–56,
        184–85
    education of, 57–58
    incorrect utilization of, 86–88, 215
    individual and organization's
        objectives, 57–58
    making improvement happen, 54
    no-layoff policy, 205
    rapid improvement circles, 74–77
    respect for, 41–42, 135, 209, 218
employer-sponsored health insurance,
    4, 13
equipment purchases, 109
"Error-Free Pathology: Applying Lean
    Production Methods to

Anatomic Pathology" (Condel, Sharbaugh, and Raab), 110, 157–90
error proofing (poka-yoke), 37, 92, 220
excess inventory, 96–99
excess processing, 100–102, 181
executive compensation, 22–27

Failure Mode and Effects Analysis (FMEA), 37–38, 71
Feeley, S., 145
Feinstein, K. W., 110
Fillingham, D., 260
financial analysts/auditors, 106
financial measures/reports, 66–67, 111
Fisher, K., 145
Fishman, C., 267
Fiume, O. J., 191
5 why's, 221
5S program (sort, set in order, shine, standardize and sustain), 80–82, 217, 219
    anatomic pathology case, 175–80
    VA Pittsburgh case study, 151–55
flowcharts, 116–17
FMEA analysis. *See* Failure Mode and Effects Analysis (FMEA)
focus groups, 46
Ford, H., 158–60, 226
Ford Motors, 7, 18–20, 39
Four Days with Dr. Deming (Deming), 5
frontline employees, 52
full-time equivalents (FTEs), 194

gain-sharing program, 78, 136
General Electric (GE), 76, 104
General Motors (GM), 5–7, 18–20
Georgetown, KY Toyota Factory case study, 267–77
Girard, M., 145
Goal, The (Goldratt), 110
Godt, L., 145
Goldratt, E. M., 63, 110–12
government intervention/relations, 15, 108–09

gross domestic product (GDP), 31
group leader, 73
group objectives, 77–78
Grunden, N., 82, 151
guided design, 71

Hammer, M., 42
health insurance
    administrative/overhead costs, 26–30, 131–32
    cost to businesses, 7–8
    GM's costs of, 5–6
    rising premiums of, 3–13
    uninsured, 13–15
healthcare
    building a safer system, 36–38
    changeover improvement process (example), 222–23
    eliminating barriers to improvement, 224–25
    fixing from inside, 229–35
    lean thinking in, 202–11, 219
    misuse of, 35
    poor quality of, 35
    quality problems in, 34–38, 231
    redesigning of, 39–41
    steps to improve, 45–46
    to-do list for national improvement, 139–41
    Toyota-like production system for, 135–38, 165–66, 191–212
    U.S. performance ranking, 32–34
healthcare alignment, 47
healthcare costs, 3, 9. *See also* lean business practice; waste
    challenges to manufacturers, 16–17
    consumer price index (CPI), 8
    excess administrative/overhead costs, 22–25
    overhead costs, 26
    as percentage of GDP, 30–32
    performance vs., 32–34
    pricelists for, 10
    reasons for escalation of, 13
    reduction of, 15–18
    typical salaries, 22–27
    U.S. per capita spending, 32–34
    waste in, 21–22

healthcare scorecard, 140
healthcare worker shortages, 16
heijunka (production leveling), 258
Hewitt Associates, 68
Hilton, D., 19
Hoglund, W., 5
hospital daily staffing report (score-
    card example), 62
"How Hospital Heal Themselves,"
    82
human resources department, 103
Humana Inc., 7, 28
hybrid health care system, 15

implementation management, 224–27
improvement goals/milestone dates,
    59–61
improvement philosophies, 72
improvement projects (*hamsei*), 80
improvement team, 67
infant mortality rate, 34
infection control nurses/staff, 105
information technology, 107–08
inspectors, 103–04
Institute for Healthcare Improvement
    (IHI), 21, 129, 191, 193, 212
Institute of Medicine (IOM), 36, 165,
    230
internal processes, 197
International Organization for
    Standardization (ISO), 128
inventory, 83, 96–99, 111, 215, 226
ISO 9000, 72, 128–29
ISO 9001 process documentation,
    112–13

Jewish Healthcare Foundation, 166
jidoka (quality in station), 89, 91–92,
    259
Jimmerson, C., 21
job classifications, 88
job rotation, 88
Joint Commission for Accreditation of
    Healthcare Organizations
    (JCAHO), 38
Jones, D., 21, 258, 260, 265
Juran, J., 46, 71
just-in-time (JIT), 53, 221, 258

kaikaku (radical improvement),
    114–15, 175, 258, 261, 263
Kaiser Family Foundation, 3
kaizen, 113–14, 161, 198, 199, 207,
    218, 254, 258
kaizen blitz, 218, 226, 258, 261
kaizen improvement team, 76
kanban system, 51, 97–99, 177, 180,
    221, 258
Kaplan, G. S., 191, 259–60
Kluger, D. M., 232
Kobayashi, I., 46, 77, 85
Kohn, L. T., 232
Krafcik, J., 21

Lagnado, L., 10–11
leadership/lean leaders, 52–54, 195,
    218
lean baseline assessment, 217
lean business practice. *See also* waste
    building blocks of, 218–22
    core concepts/key precepts of,
        195–97, 225–27, 258–60,
        263
    critics of, 263–65
    description of, 214–15
    evolution of, 158–59, 227–28
    getting started with, 197–202
    in healthcare, 213–27
    starting point for, 216–22
    as winning strategy, 214
lean enterprise, 198, 223–24
Lean Enterprise Institute, 20–21
lean production, 8, 15–16, 20–22, 42,
    45, 161. *See also* Toyota Lean
    Production System (TPS),
    anatomic pathology case, 157–90
    building blocks of, 217
    defined, 20, 22
    implementation of, 50–51
    lean leaders, 52–54
    reasons for, 17–18
    Toyota Lean Production, 18–21
lean thinking, 192
Lean Thinking (Womack and Jones),
    21, 258
Leape, L., 230
learning line, 167–75, 234
legal counsel, 106

LifeCare Hospitals, 244
Liker, J. K., 163, 164, 276

McCalister, M. B., 7
McCray, E., 82, 151
Machine That Changed the World, The
     (Womack), 97, 161
magnet hospital environment/shared
     governance, 119
Makl, D. G., 232
management by sight, 83–85
managers, 52–54, 103–05, 136, 224,
     227
"Manufacturing in America—A
     Comprehensive Strategy to
     Address the Challenges to U.S.
     Manufacturers" (U.S. Dept. of
     Commerce), 16
manufacturing companies, 159–61
marketing, 106
mass training, 217
medical bankruptcies, 15
medical errors, 36–37, 165, 230,
     232–33, 236–37
Medical Savings Insurance Company
     of Oklahoma and Indiana, 40
Medicare compliance officers/staff,
     106
Medicare/Medicaid, 13, 26, 32, 40,
     133
medication administration, 247–48
meetings, 101
Midwest Business Group on Health
     (MBGH), 13, 34–35
Miller, D., 191
model line approach, 249–53
Monongahela Valley Hospital, 244
monopoly power, 9, 16
Moreland, M., 82, 151
motion, 94–96, 215
muda (waste), 21, 193, 198, 258

National Committee for Quality
     Assurance (NCQA), 140–41
National Health Service (NHS) (case
     study), 257–65
     Bolton Hospitals Trust, 260–61
     kaizen blitz, 261

     lean thinking and, 260–61
     lessons of, 261–63
national healthcare expenditure,
     30–31
national healthcare policy, 15, 140
National Institute of Standards and
     Technology Manufacturing
     Extension Partnership
     (NIST/MEP), 213
NUMMI (New United Motor
     Manufacturing, Inc.) plant,
     73–74, 78, 88, 91, 161
"Nun and the Bureaucrat, The," 82
nursing care delivery models, 119–20
nursing homes, 133

obesity epidemic, 34
Ohno, T., 41, 46, 85, 91, 97, 109,
     159–60, 181, 227, 258
O'Neill, P., 132, 165
operating expense, 111
organizational capabilities, 234
organizational structure for
     quality/cost improvement, 58,
     66, 77, 203
overhead costs, 22–30
overproduction/wrong product, 85–86,
     100–102, 181, 215
overstaffing/understaffing, 86

Pareto fashion, 61
partners, 120–21, 138
pathology errors, 166
patient advocate, 104–05
patient care paths, 51
patient care received, 35–36
patient experience, 60
patient-focused care, 119–20
patient lawsuits, 106
patient value added (PVA), 46–48, 59,
     116–17
Perfecting Patient Care (PPC) System,
     166
performance measures
     continuous flow and, 110–11, 202
     financial indicators, 111
Perreiah, P., 153
personal bankruptcies, 15

personal healthcare expenditures, 30
Physician's Clinic of Iowa (PCI), 113
Pittsburgh Regional Healthcare
    Initiative (PRHI) case study, 82,
    165–66, 242–45, 246
plan, do, check, act methodology, 71,
    199, 202, 226
point of use storage (POUS), 220
poka-yoke techniques, 37, 92, 220
prescription drugs, 30, 68–69, 133
price lists, 10–11
PricewaterhouseCoopers, 3
primary processes, 197
primary/total nursing care, 119
problem-solving methodology, 71, 79
process cycle times, 117–18
process flowchart, 112
process improvement methods, 45,
    177, 196–97, 240
"Psychology of Change Management"
    (*McKinsey Quarterly*), 55–56
pull system, 51, 148, 213, 217, 222,
    263

quality, defined, 20
quality circles, 75
Quality and Cost Improvement
    Council, 57, 59, 68, 80
Quality and Cost Improvement
    Department, 56–57
Quality and Cost Improvement
    Manual, 57, 79, 113
quality improvement, 15–18
    at the source, 221
    organizational structure for, 58, 77
    past failures of, 38–39
quality reports, 66–67
quality in station, 137
queuing situations, 61
quick changeover, 118, 137, 220

Raab, S. S., 110, 157
radical improvement, 114–15
Rapid Improvement Circles (RICs),
    57, 66, 74–77, 115, 136
Rapid Improvement Events (RIEs),
    54, 76

Rapid Improvement Team (RIT), 57,
    66–70, 74–77, 136
    Toyota-style work teams, 70–74
Rapid Process Improvement Weeks
    (RPIW), 195
Rapid Process Improvements (RPIs),
    76
    Children's Hospital case study,
    145–50
recognition program, 55, 79, 136
red-tag holding area, 83
reengineering, 41–42
regional centers, 39
"respect for humanity" principle, 41,
    209
rewards, 55, 78–79, 136
reworks, 88–83
risk priority number (RPN), 38
root-cause analyses, 92

safety/risk managers/staff, 106
satellite centers, 39
scheduling system, 51
Schwarzenegger, A., 26
scorecard, 61–63
    for department monitoring, 63–65
    for entire organization, 61–63
Scotchmer, A., 257
secretarial staff, 107
SEIU District 1199 union, 11
sequencing work, 109, 137
Sharbaugh, D. T., 110, 157
Shingo, S., 46, 227
Shinjijutsu International Centre, 259
Shook, J., 277
simulation and experimentation,
    245–49
Sisters of Mary Health Care
    (SSMHC), 127
Six Layers of Resistance to buy-in,
    55–56
Six Sigma, 71, 92, 93, 157, 216
"Small Improvements Yield Big
    Results in Shadyside Pathology
    Lab," 110
Social Security, 32
spaghetti diagram, 117
Spear, S., 162, 171, 229, 270
staff. *See* Employees

stakeholders, 67
standardization, 81, 109–10, 114, 137,
   152, 217, 220
strategic plan
   improvement plan and, 59–61
   quality/cost improvement goals,
      65–66
strategic quality/cost improvement
   goals, 65–66
sunset date, 66
supervisors, 52–54, 103–05
suppliers, 120–21, 138, 220
surveys, 46
system errors, 162

Takt time, 84, 222
team charter, 102
team leader and members, 70–75,
   136, 167
team/functional nursing care, 119
ThedaCare, Inc. case study, 207–11
Theory of Constraints, 55
Thomas, E. J., 232
throughput, 111
*To Err Is Human: Building a Safer
   Health System* (IOM), 36, 165
total productive maintenance (TPM),
   222
total quality management (TQM), 214
   past failures of, 38–39
total systems view, 132–33
Toussaint, J., 191
Toyoda family, 158–59, 227
Toyota Lean Production System
   (TPS), 18–21, 41, 46, 72,
   79–80, 157, 192
   background to, 158–65, 227–28
   built-in quality, 20
   Georgetown, KY case study,
      267–77
   healthcare application (summary),
      135–38
   just-in-time production/inventory,
      20
   people-work connection, 162
   principles of, 163–64
   respect for employee, 20
   three pillars of, 20
   total systems view, 132–33

Toyota Motor Company, 18–20, 45,
   158–65
Toyota-style work teams, 70–74
*Toyota Way: 14 Management
   Principles from the World's
   Greatest Manufacturer* (Liker),
   163–64, 276
transportation waste, 47, 94–95, 181,
   215
20 Keys to Workplace Improvement
   (Kobayashi), 77, 85
"Twice the Price—What Uninsured
   and Under Insured Patients Pay
   for Hospital Care" (Care for
   Ohio), 11

uninsured population, 13–15
United Auto Workers Union, 6
United Healthcare, 28
"U.S. Firms Losing Health Care
   Battle, GM Chairman Says," 6
U.S. per capita spending on health-
   care, 32–34
United Way Organization, 141
universal healthcare system, 29–30
University of Pittsburgh School of
   Medicine (UPMC), 166, 244,
   246, 249
unnecessary motion, 94–96, 215
utilization review staff, 104

VA Pittsburgh Health System, 151–55
value, 263
   definition of, 46
value-added tasks, 46, 197, 213
value alignment, 42
value stream, 47, 193, 197, 220, 263
value-stream map, 47–48, 200–201,
   217
videotaping work processes, 115–16
Virginia Mason Medical Center case
   example, 194–95, 202–07, 253,
   259–60
visual control, 63, 83–85, 176, 179,
   217, 243
visual workplace, 138, 219
Voluntary Hospital Association
   (VHA), 140

Wagoner, G. R., Jr., 6–7
waits and delays, 50, 93–94, 215
waste, 35, 41, 85, 215–16
    bureaucratic layers, 103–08
    causes and variation of, 216
    correction of, 93
    defects and rework, 88–93
    elimination of, 85–102, 137, 181
    excess inventory, 96–99
    excess processing, 100–101
    government relations area, 108–09
    incorrect utilization of staff,
        86–88
    information technology area,
        107–08
    overproduction/wrong product,
        85–86
    potential waste areas, 103–09
    transportation, 94
    unnecessary motion, 94–96
    waits and delays, 93–94
    work-arounds, 168, 235–37, 238,
        241

Web sites, 108
Welch, J., 104
Western Pennsylvania Hospital case
    study, 237–42
Wisconsin Hospital Association
    (WHA), 13
Wolk, K., 165
Womack, J. P., 21, 46, 97, 103, 191,
    258
Woodward, G. A., 145
work-arounds as waste, 168, 235–37,
    238, 241
work-out groups, 76
work pace (*takt* time), 84, 222
work sequence, 84, 109–10
work teams, 73, 75
work zones, 147
workplace layout, 219
World Health Organization (WHO),
    31–32

zero-tolerance, 105